Nerve Agents Poisoning and its Treatment in Schematic Figures and Tables

T0297344

Nerve Agents Poisoning and its Treatment in Schematic Figures and Tables

Jiri Bajgar

Department of Toxicology
Faculty of Military Health Sciences
University of Defence
Hradec Kralove

and

Department of Radiology and Toxicology
Faculty of Social and Health Studies
University of South Bohemia
Ceske Budějovice
Czech Republic

AMSTERDAM • BOSTON • HEIDELBERG • LONDON • NEW YORK • OXFORD • PARIS
SAN DIEGO • SAN FRANCISCO • SINGAPORE • SYDNEY • TOKYO

ELSEVIER

Elsevier
32 Jamestown Road, London NW1 7BY
225 Wyman Street, Waltham, MA 02451, USA

First edition 2012

Notices
Knowledge and best practice in this field are constantly changing. As new research and experience broaden our understanding, changes in research methods, professional practices, or medical treatment may become necessary.

Practitioners and researchers must always rely on their own experience and knowledge in evaluating and using any information, methods, compounds, or experiments described herein. In using such information or methods they should be mindful of their own safety and the safety of others, including parties for whom they have a professional responsibility.

To the fullest extent of the law, neither the Publisher nor the authors, contributors, or editors, assume any liability for any injury and/or damage to persons or property as a matter of products liability, negligence or otherwise, or from any use or operation of any methods, products, instructions, or ideas contained in the material herein.

British Library Cataloguing-in-Publication Data
A catalogue record for this book is available from the British Library

Library of Congress Cataloging-in-Publication Data
A catalog record for this book is available from the Library of Congress

ISBN: 978-0-323-28249-9

For information on all Elsevier publications
visit our website at elsevierdirect.com

This book has been manufactured using Print On Demand technology. Each copy is produced to order and is limited to black ink. The online version of this book will show color figures where appropriate.

Working together to grow
libraries in developing countries

www.elsevier.com | www.bookaid.org | www.sabre.org

ELSEVIER   BOOK AID International   Sabre Foundation

Contents

Acknowledgments

This work was supported by the Grant FVZ 0000501. Correction of the English by Mrs. E. Drahokoupilova is gratefully acknowledged. Last but not least, I thank my wife, Jitka, for her love and understanding lasting more than 50 years.

1 Introduction

In the group of organophosphates (OPs), nerve agents are considered the most important chemical warfare agents (CWAs). They are an integral part of chemical weapons (CWs). These highly toxic chemicals represent potential threats to civilian populations, as evident from terrorist attacks in Japan in the 1990s. Therefore, research on their effect, diagnosis, treatment, and prophylaxis of intoxication by these compounds has been one of the main topics within the programs of various laboratories.

OP nerve agents are inhibitors of cholinesterase. Beyond this main pharmacological property, they have many other effects that involve the activation of multiple noncholinergic neurotransmitter systems in the central nervous system: mutagenic, stressogenic, immunotoxic, hepatotoxic, membraneous, and hematotoxic, depending on the type of compound. Nerve agent–induced effects are usually manifested immediately after high-level or intermediate-level exposures to these CWAs. Nevertheless, numerous studies of both humans and other animals show that survivors of high-level and possibly intermediate-level exposure to nerve agents can experience subtle but significant long-term neurological and neuropsychological outcomes that are detectable months or even years after the recovery from acute poisoning. Thus, exposure to nerve agents leading to acute effects or chronic exposure to nerve agents may well lead to delayed and persistent adverse effects, mostly neuropsychological.

All of these features document that nerve agents act on the nervous systems, both central and peripheral, and affect cholinergic nerve transmission. However, the cholinergic nervous system is not isolated; it is related to other nerve transmitters and neuromodulators. Therefore, our knowledge of dealing with the action of nerve agents and protecting against them is a significant contribution to neuropharmacology, neurophysiology, and toxicology in general. Although different books already deal with these topics, they are too specialized and do not give a simple and quick overview of the problem.

The current book attempts to summarize some recent results—in simple forms, mostly in schematic figures and tables—with the aim of facilitating research work in this field for those who are beginning these studies.

Nerve Agents Poisoning and its Treatment in Schematic Figures and Tables. DOI: 10.1016/B978-0-12-416047-7.00001-3

2 Chemical Weapons

As weapons of mass destruction, the ban of CWs was discussed at the Conference on Disarmament (CD) in Geneva. The text of future conventions dealing with CWs was successfully elaborated, and the CWC was signed in Paris in 1993. The CWC entered into force on April 29, 1997, just 180 days after ratification by 65 states who were party to the convention. More than 60% of CW stocks were destroyed. Currently, 188 state parties (and two signatories) are involved. The use of CWs or highly toxic chemicals has not been entirely prevented; terrorists in Japan in 1994 and 1995, for example, used one CW to deadly effect.

As a unique international document, the CWC eliminates one type of weapon of mass destruction under strict international control. The document contains more than 200 pages with 24 articles and annexes. The preamble (printed as follows in bold italics) specifically cites herbicides as potential CWs:

Preamble

—Recognizing the prohibition, embodied in the pertinent agreements and relevant principles of international law, of the use of herbicides as a method of warfare,—

Article I—General obligations: (a basic sense of the convention is formulated)

1. *Each State Party to this Convention undertakes never under any circumstances: to develop, produce, otherwise acquire, stockpile or retain chemical weapons, or transfer, directly or indirectly, chemical weapons to anyone;*
   The text also contains the restriction about not using CWs:
   ... to use chemical weapons;
   This article also obliges signatories to destroy CWs and their production facilities:
2. *Each State Party undertakes to destroy chemical weapons ....*
4. *Each State Party undertakes to destroy any chemical weapons production facilities ...,*
   Simultaneously, the article prohibits the use of riot-control agents for military purposes:
5. *Each State Party undertakes not to use riot control agents as a method of warfare.*
   Article II then specifies exactly what chemical weapons are.

Article II—Definitions and Criteria

1. *"Chemical weapons" means the following, together or separately:*
   a. *Toxic chemicals and their precursors, except where intended for purposes not prohibited under this Convention, as long as the types and quantities are consistent with such purposes;*
   b. *Munitions and devices, specifically designed to cause death or other harm through the toxic properties of those toxic chemicals specified in subparagraph (a), which would be released as a result of the employment of such munitions and devices;*
   c. *Any equipment specifically designed for use directly in connection with the employment of munitions and devices specified in subparagraph (b).*

   Then the next paragraph defines toxic chemicals.

Nerve Agents Poisoning and its Treatment in Schematic Figures and Tables. DOI: 10.1016/B978-0-12-416047-7.00002-5

2. *"Toxic chemical" means:*

Any chemical which through its chemical action on life processes can cause death, temporary incapacitation or permanent harm to humans or animals. This includes all such chemicals, regardless of their origin or their method of production, and regardless of whether they are produced in facilities, in munitions or elsewhere.

Thus, a CWA can be characterized as a toxic chemical.

To develop effective countermeasures against the effects of nerve agents, the convention contains the following article:

Article VI—Activities not prohibited under this Convention—allowing to develop, produce, otherwise acquire, retain, transfer and use of toxic chemicals and their precursors for purposes not prohibited under this Convention. However, these activities are to be declared and controlled.

Conclusions

Although the CWC is functioning well, it does not cover terrorist activities connected with the use of CWs and thus their use is not excluded.

3 Chemical Warfare Agents

There are different groups of CWAs. They can be divided into two types: those used against humans and those used against plants. The second group is not included in the CWC schedules; it is generally covered in the CWC's preamble.

CWA use against humans can be characterized as lethal (causing death) or incapacitant (causing physical or psychical incapacitation) (Figure 3.1).

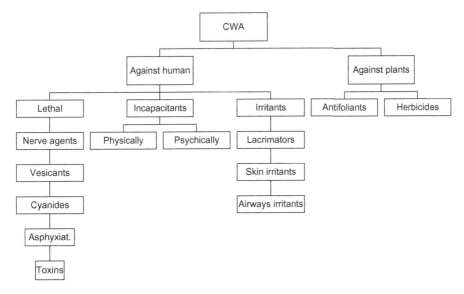

Figure 3.1 Classification of CWAs.

Nerve Agents Poisoning and its Treatment in Schematic Figures and Tables. DOI: 10.1016/B978-0-12-416047-7.00003-7

4 Organophosphates and Nerve Agents

Organic phosphates play important roles in living organisms—e.g., in photosynthesis, metabolic pathways, synthetic reactions, nucleic acids, coenzyme systems, and transmission of signals. They are involved in energetic metabolism and influence the action of hormones or neuromediators. Chemically synthesized organic compounds of phosphorus show a broad variety of biological properties. Very important chemicals in this group are organophosphorus inhibitors of cholinesterases (commonly called OPs).

These compounds produce acute effects that are characterized by their influence on cholinergic nerve transmission. Some of them (nerve agents) can be and have been misused as CWs by military forces and by terrorists, even though an international convention prohibits their misuse. Figure 4.1 briefly summarizes possible exposures to these toxic chemicals. Simultaneously, biological weapons are prohibited by another international convention: the Convention on the Prohibition of the Development, Production, and Stockpiling of Bacteriological (Biological) and Toxic Weapons and on Their Destruction (which became effective in March 1975). The basic elements (Articles) of these two Conventions are given in Figures 4.2 and 4.3.

Although these two conventions have a similar aim (to eliminate one type of weapon of mass destruction), there are differences between them, mostly dealing with control of their implementation (Table 4.1).

The development of the CWC was difficult and was not finalized until the 1990s. The CWC entered into force on April 29, 1997 after ratification by 65 nations. Twelve countries have declared OP CW factories where CWs were made after January 1, 1946 (Bosnia and Herzegovina, China, France, Iran, Japan, Serbia and Montenegro, United Kingdom, India, Libya, Russia, South Korea, and United States of America). The last five countries have declared possession of CWs; possession (but without manufacturing factories) has been also declared by Albania. Table 4.2 shows some of the milestones in the use of toxic chemicals and negotiations on the ban of their military use. Clearly, nerve agents are the most important.

This book is focused on the description of the action of OP and nerve agents and principles of diagnosis, prophylaxis, and treatment. Their action was described in many publications, beginning with Koelle (1963) and finishing with Gupta (2009). For simplification, tables and schematic figures provide most of the relevant information; the use of references is limited (some references for more detailed information are mentioned in the chapter References, Further reading).

A large variety of compounds with different physical, chemical, and biological properties, including toxicity, can be observed in the OP group. OPs differ in their toxicity from practically nontoxic (e.g., malathion) to highly toxic (e.g., nerve

Nerve Agents Poisoning and its Treatment in Schematic Figures and Tables. DOI: 10.1016/B978-0-12-416047-7.00004-9

Production, processing, storing, transport
(either for intentional or unintentional use)
↓
Use, release

Intentional	**Unintentional**
↓	↓
Terrorism or sabotage	Natural disaster (H_2S and others), coincidence of
military or local conflict	conditions, technical fault or failure of human factor
(CWA, other toxic chemicals)	(toxic industrial chemicals, CWA, precursors etc.)

Figure 4.1 The possibilities of exposure to toxic chemicals.

Preamble
Art. I—definitions, not to develop, produce,
           othervise acquire, stockpile, transfer
Art. II—destruction of BW
Art. III—transfer
Art. IV—national laws
Art. V—consultation, redress a situation
Art. VI—facts findings
Art. VII—assistance (use or threat of use of BW)
Art. VIII—relation to GP 25
Art. IX—CWC
Art. X—exchange of science and technology information
Art. XI—changes
Art. XII—review conferences
Art. XIII—duration
Art. XIV—signing, ratification (22)
Art. XV—language, depositary

Figure 4.2 Biological Weapons Convention (BWC) articles: Convention on the Prohibition of the Development, Production and Stockpiling of Bacteriological (Biological) and Toxin Weapons and on Their Destruction entered into force in March 1975.

agents). The component chemicals are available for benign chemical syntheses, and starting materials and methods for nerve agents synthesis are easily acquired. The most important group having a significant biological effect includes compounds of the general formula.

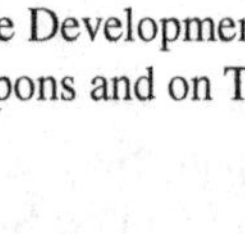

$$R^1—\overset{\overset{\displaystyle R^2}{|}}{\underset{\underset{\displaystyle O}{||}}{P}}—R^3$$

where R^1 and R^2 are hydrogen, alkyl (including cyclic), aryl and others, alkoxy, alkylthio, and amino groups. R^3 is a dissociable group (e.g., halogens, cyano, alkylthio group, rest of inorganic or organic acid). More on the chemistry of these compounds is given by Fest and Schmidt (1982).

Preamble
Art. I—general obligations (+use)
Art. II—definitions and criteria
Art. III—declarations
Art. IV—chemical weapons
Art. V—CW production facilities
Art. VI—activities not prohibited under this Convention
Art. VII—national implementation measures
Art. VIII—the Organization
Art. IX—consultation, cooperation, fact-finding
Art. X—assistance and protection
Art. XI—economic and technological development
Art. XII—to redress a situation including sanctions
Art. XIII—relation to other agreements
Art. XIV—settlement of disputes
Art. XV—amendments
Art. XVI—duration and withdrawal
Art. XVII—status of the Annexes
Art. XVIII—signature
Art. XIX—ratification
Art. XX—accession
Art. XXI—entry into force (65)
Art. XXII—reservations
Art. XXIII—depositary
Art. XXIV—authentic texts
Annex on Chemicals
Annex on Implementation and Verification ("Verification Annex")
Annex on the Protection of Confidential Information ("Confidentiality Annex")

Figure 4.3 CWC articles: Convention on the Prohibition of the Development, Production, Stockpiling, and Use of Chemical Weapons and on Their Destruction entered into force in April 1997.

Table 4.1 Differences and Similarities Between the BWC and the CWC

Problem	BWC	CWC
Entry into force: scope	Yes	Yes
Prohibition of research	No	No
Prohibition of development	Yes	Yes
Prohibition of production	Yes	Yes
Prohibition of acquisition	Yes	Yes
Prohibition of transfer	Yes	Yes
Prohibition of storage	Yes	Yes
Prohibition of use	No[a]	Yes
Destruction of stocks	Yes	Yes
Destruction of production facilities	No	Yes
International organization inspectorate	No	Yes
Formal declaration of weapons	No	Yes
Formal declaration of production facilities	No	Yes
Formal declaration of unprohibited activities	No	Yes
Confidence-building measures (CBMs)	Yes	No[b]

[a]Discussed; generally it is accepted that the use of biological weapons is prohibited because the BWC exists, although no article in the BWC prohibits such use.
[b]CBMs are voluntary; they do not exist as such in the CWC. Declarations contain similar information and are therefore more or less equal to CBMs.

Table 4.2 Some Milestones Related to Use/Release of Toxic Chemicals

Year(s)	Event
2000 BC	Toxic smokes in China induce sleep
Fourth century BC	Spartakus: toxic smokes
184 BC	Hannibal: baskets with poisonous snakes
1168	Fustat (Cairo): use of Greek fire
1422	Bohemia region: cesspools (H_2S)
1456	Beograde: rats with arsenic
Nineteenth century	Admiral Dundonald: proposed use of chemicals in war
1914–1918	World War I: birth of chemical war
1918–1939	Development of new CWs and protective means
June 17, 1925	Geneva Protocol
December 23, 1936	Lange and Kruger: synthesis of tabun
1940–1945	Concentration camps: cyanides
1943	Synthesis of sarin
1943	Hoffmann and Stoll: synthesis of LSD-25
1945	Kuhn: synthesis of soman
1950	V agents are developed
1961–1968	Production of VX
1962	BZ introduced into military arsenals
1970	Bicycle phosphates considered as potential CWAs
1976	Seveso: release of dioxin
1980	Rumors of intermediate volatility agent
1984	Bhopal incident: release of methylisocyanate
1985	Decision on production of binary CWs
1986, 1987	Demonstration of US CWs (Tooele) and Soviet CWs (Shikhany) to the CD in Geneva
1987	Production of binary CWs
1988	Halabja: use of mustard
1980–1990	Rumors of new nerve agent Novichok
1989	Conference in Paris on chemical disarmament
1991	Persian Gulf War: veteran's syndrome
1992	BZ military stocks of the United States destroyed
1992	Geneva: finalization of the rolling text of the CWC at the CD
1993	Signing CWC in Paris
1993	Preparatory commission on OP CWs
1994	CWs of Iraq destroyed
1994	Aum Shinrikyo: sarin attack in Matsumoto
1995	Aum Shinrikyo: sarin attak in Tokyo
April 29, 1997	CWC enters into force; OP CW established in The Hague
2000	Research on nonlethal weapons intensified
2002	Moscow threatens fentanyl derivatives used against terrorists
29 April 2012	CW of the State Parties to the CWC will be destroyed (it is prolonged)

Source: Reprinted from Gupta (2009) with permission.

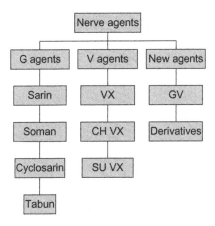

Figure 4.4 Classification of nerve agents.

Table 4.3 LD$_{50}$ Values of GV in Mice and Rats with Various Routes of Administration

$$CH_3-N(CH_3)-P(=O)(F)-CH_2CH_2N(CH_3)-CH_3$$

Routes of Administration	Mice	Rats
	LD$_{50}$ (μg/kg) with Their 95% Confidence Limits	
IV	27.6 (25.6–29.4)	11 (8.5–17.6)
IM	30.5 (28–55)	17 (15.5–23.6)
SC	32 (29–53)	21 (18–26)
PO	222 (194–255)	190 (881–272)
PC	Not tested	1,366 (881–3,138)

Nerve agents differ in chemical structure and are divided into G and V agents. New groups of nerve agents are represented by chemicals containing radicals of G and V agents (GV or GP agents) in their structure. Schematic representation of the groups of nerve agents is given in Figure 4.4. General formulas and toxicities of some GV agents are given in Table 4.3. Physicochemical properties of selected nerve agents are given in Table 4.4. Chemical formulas of some OP nerve agents are demonstrated in Figure 4.5, and toxicities for rats and extrapolated values for humans are shown in Table 4.5.

The toxicity depends on the route of administration. The highest toxicity is observed for intravenous (IV) administration; it is given by direct administration of

Table 4.4 Physical Chemical Properties of Selected Nerve Agents

Agent	Molecular Weight	Specific Gravity	Melting Point	Boiling Point	Volatility
Tabun, GA	162.3	1.073	−49	246	611
Sarin, GB	140.1	1.009	−56	147	21,862
Soman, GD	182.18	1.022	−80	167	3,921
VX	267.36	1.008	−20	300	10.7
GV (GP)	198.18	1.11	0	207–240	700
Cyclosarin, GF	180.14	1.133	−12	239	659 (581)

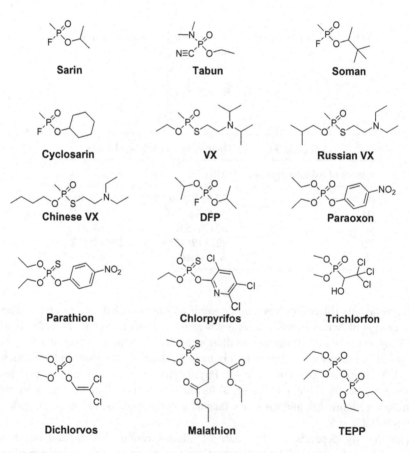

Figure 4.5 Structures of some organophosphorus cholinesterase inhibitors.

Table 4.5 Toxicities for Rats (Experimentally Determined) and Humans (Assessed) for different OPs and Nerve Agents

Compound and Synonyms	Toxicity (LD$_{50}$)			
	[a]IM, Rat (μg/kg)	[a]PO, Rat (mg/kg)	[b]PO, Human (mg/kg)	[c]IM, Human (μg/kg)
VX	14 (8–16)	0.085 (0.08–0.09)	0.07	22.5 (20–25)
Sarin 113, Trilon 46, T-144, IMPF, GB	200	0.8 (0.7–0.9)	0.14 (0.11–0.17)	–
Soman, GD, PMFP	70	0.55 (0.5–0.6)	13.5 (0.1–0.17)	–
GV, GP, EA 5365, IVA	17	0.19	0.11	22.5 (20–25)
DFP	800	7 (1–13)	0.7 (0.29–1.1)	45 (40–50)
TEPP, Tetron	850	8.5 (2–15)	0.93 (0.43–1.43)	–
Paraoxon, E 600, Mintacol	400 (300–500)	3	0.57 (0.43–0.71)	325 (300–350)
Parathion, E 605, Bladan, Alkron, Folidol, Tiofos, Niran, Rhodiatox	700 (500–900)	6.5 (6–7)	1.79 (0.71–2.86)	2,900 (2,800–3,000)
Dichlorvos, DDVP	17,440	62	10.7 (7.14–14.29)	175 (150–200)
Trichlorfon, Chlorofos, Phospchlor, Trichlorfos, Metriphonate, Dipterex, Dylox, Neguvon, Tugon	230,000	625	250 (100–400)	–
Systox	3,110	11.5 (9–14)	0.86 (0.29–1.43)	4,000
Dimethoate, Bopardoil, Cygon Daphene, Fostion MM, Perfekthion, Phosphamid, Rogor, Roxion, Dimethoate Bayer	1,500	242.5 (215–270)	21.5 (14.3–28.6)	1,500
Chlorfenvinfos, Birlan, Dermaton, Supona	5,000	15	1.0 (0.571–1.4286)	2,500
Dicrotofos, Bidrin, Carbicron	8,500 (7–10,000)	22	2.145 (1.43–2.86)	–
Diazinon, Basudin, Exudin, Sarolex	65,000 (50–80,000)	125 (100–150)	13.6 (10–17.1)	–
Fosfamidon, Dimecron, Dixon	12,500 (10–15,000	27.5	2.0 (1.43–2.57)	8,500
Malathion, Karbofos	–	1,000 (800–1,200)	70 (40–100)	–

(Continued)

Table 4.5 (Continued)

Compound and Synonyms	Toxicity (LD$_{50}$)			
	[a]IM, Rat (μg/kg)	[a]PO, Rat (mg/kg)	[b]PO, Human (mg/kg)	[c]IM, Human (μg/kg)
Et-Met, 25SN, Medemo, EDMM	28.9	0.121	0.11	3.5
iPr–iPr	46	0.056	0.02	6.5
Et–Et, VM, edemo	20	0.212	0.04	12
iPr–Met	96	0.874	0.1	14
Russian VX, RVX	14.1	0.02	–	32.3

Source: Modified from Bajgar (2004).
[a]Experimental data from literature (different sources—e.g., Bajgar (2004, 2005)).
[b]Assessed data, literature sources (Bajgar, 2004; Gupta, 2009; Marrs et al., 1996).
[c]Assessed data using extrapolation (Bajgar, 2004, 2009).

Table 4.6 Toxicities of Selected Nerve Agents for Mice Determined as LD$_{50}$ (mg/kg) at IV Administration at Our Department in 2010

ROA	Tabun	Sarin	Soman	VX
IV	0.15 (0.11–0.19)	0.143 (0.127–0.160)	0.076 (0.07–0.082)	0.0145 (0.012–0.017)
IM	0.275 (0.269–0.281)	0.215 (0.193–0.238)	0.124 (0.106–0.145)	0.0268 (0.0264–0.0273)
SC	0.3	0.252 (0.241–0.246)	0.15 (0.129–0.179)	–
IP	0.6	0.4 (0.346–0.462)	0.24 (0.218–0.264)	0.0442 (0.037–0.054)
PO	–	1.019 (0.893–1.168)	1.614 (1.365–1.908)	–

In addition, available toxicities at other routes of administration are given.

the agent into the bloodstream, and all its losses during penetration through biological barriers are excluded. The toxicities of three nerve agents (LD$_{50}$, IV) for mice are given in Table 4.6, including 95% confidence limits demonstrating statistical error for this determination.

At the most obvious routes of administration, the toxicity is usually decreased (as LD$_{50}$ value) in the order from intramuscular (IM) < subcutaneous (SC) < oral (PO) < percutaneous (PC), although exceptions exist. This increase is of similar character for IM, SC, intraperitoneal (IP), and PO administration for all studied nerve agents (Figure 4.6). Toxicities of some OPs and nerve agents are shown in Table 4.7.

The PC administration has another characteristic probably caused by more complicated penetration from the skin to target organs. Some toxicities are demonstrated

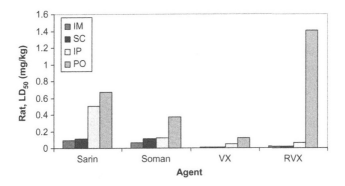

Figure 4.6 Toxicities of selected nerve agents at various routes of administration.

Table 4.7 Toxicities of Some Nerve Agents and OPs in Rats at Different Routes of Administration (LD$_{50}$, mg/kg)

Agent	IM	SC	IP	PO	PC
Tabun	0.183	0.27	0.56–0.6	3.6	400
Sarin	0.096–0.2	0.11	0.47–0.5	0.67	117.9
Soman	0.069	0.11–0.12	0.117	0.37	9.987
VX	0.0082	0.0119	0.0456	0.12–0.19	0.085–0.150
RVX	0.014–0.015	0.0159	0.063	1.402	0.39–0.5
GV	0.14–0.17	–	–	0.19	1.366
Paraoxon	0.321	0.429	1.276	2.519	4.4–12.1
DFP	1.399	1.58	3.2	3.33	300–400

Table 4.8 Percutaneous Toxicity of Nerve Agents in Rats

Agent	LD$_{50}$ (mg/kg)
Sarin	117.9
Soman	9.9
Tabun	400
VX	0.08
RVX	0.29
GV	1.37

LD$_{50}$, PC, guinea pig, soman—8.94; VX—0.240 mg/kg.

in Table 4.8. It can be optimized before each experiment either to determine the toxicity (maybe in two to three doses) or to compare the obtained results. Table 4.9 shows variations in toxicities with toxicity data obtained for nerve agents and rodents (rats and mice) over 20 years.

Determining inhalation toxicity is more difficult and requires special equipment that allows quantitative dosing of nerve agent vapors. Figure 4.7 shows an example

Table 4.9 Toxicities (IM) for Different Nerve Agents in Mice and
Rats Expressed as LD_{50} (µg/kg, IM) in Period 1992–2011; Means
and Variations (min−max)

Nerve Agent	Mice (1996–2011)	Rats (1992–2010)
VX	25 (16–38)	15 (8–28)
GV	30.5 (18–65)	17 (9–31)
Soman	111.9 (60–150)	78.7 (51–102)
Sarin	170.3 (120–241)	129.7 (100–180)
Cyclosarin	190 (155–232)	80 (62–103)
Tabun	275 (211–301)	168 (102–201)

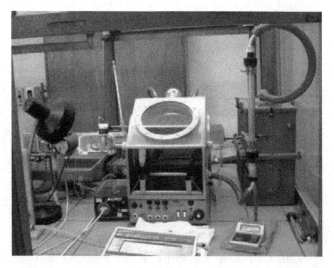

Figure 4.7 Dynamic flow inhalation chamber used in the department of toxicology, allowing
quantitative dosing of nerve agents.

of an inhalation chamber. Inhalation toxicity expressed as an LCt_{50} value is mostly
known for volatile nerve agents such as sarin and soman. Moreover, the determination
is complicated by the experimental design (the use of open or closed system, nose or
whole body exposure, time of exposure, etc.) and therefore comparison of different
values is difficult. Using our methodical approach (dynamic flow chamber), the LCt_{50}
in rats (60-min exposure) for soman was determined to be 4.1 mg/60 min/m³, and the
same value for sarin was 6.3 mg/60 min/m³. The same values for sarin for 10 min of
exposure (in mg/m³) are reported for mice (380), rats (231), rabbits (115), cats (79),
and monkeys (74) (Marrs et al., 1996).

All these data *in vivo* for animals can be compared and correlated with the constants *in vitro* obtained for human material and serve as basic information for assess-
ing nerve agent toxicity for humans. This assessment is difficult but can be simply
related to acetylcholinesterase (AChE, EC 3.1.1.7) inhibition (preferably in the

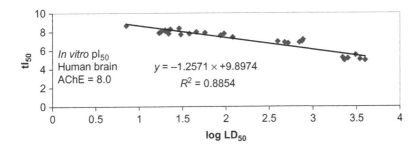

Figure 4.8 Correlation between anticholinesterase efficacy *in vitro* and toxicity *in vivo* for some V agents.

brain) *in vitro*. The affinity *in vitro* can be correlated with toxicity *in vivo* (although complicated by the route of administration; optimal is parenteral administration to minimize penetration into the blood vessel). From the regression line, toxicity can be calculated for humans, but it is a rough and orientational assessment. Figure 4.8 shows an example of this extrapolation; it is better to use agents not detoxifying in the organism, therefore the group of V agents was used. The inhibition efficacy *in vitro* for human brain AChE is given and can be extrapolated to the toxicity for humans *in vivo*.

Conclusions

OPs include compounds of different toxicities; nerve agents can be the most highly toxic chemicals with a low evaluation in civilian practice. They represent real threats (both military and terrorist) to human population; therefore, medical protection against these agents is needed.

5 Toxicodynamics

The mechanism of action (toxicodynamics) of OPs is based on irreversible AChE inhibition at the cholinergic synapses. Under normal conditions, acetylcholine forms from acetate and coenzyme A (Figure 5.1). This reaction is catalyzed by enzyme choline acetyltransferase (EC 2.3.1.6). When a signal is transmitted, a quantum of acetylcholine stored in synaptic vesicles is released to the synaptic cleft where it binds to the acetylcholine receptor; there exist minimally muscarinic and nicotinic receptors (and their subtypes). The muscarinic receptor belongs to the metabotrophic G-protein–coupled receptors family. Five subtypes (M1–M5) have been recognized. The nicotinic receptors are ligand-gated ion channels comprising usually five units.

After binding to the receptor, the receptor changes its conformation to allow an imbalance of ions and signal transmission. A schematic representation of this action is shown in Figure 5.2. This reaction in quite another picture is demonstrated in Figure 5.3.

To block action of acetylcholine after this reaction, a released neuromediator is hydrolyzed by AChE. In Figure 5.1, theoretical possibilities for influencing acetylcholine level are given. This can be caused by one change of one of the three macromolecules giving basically 81 (84 − 3 normal) possibilities. A combination of changes of two or all three macromolecules is possible but not calculated. Because of AChE inhibition, acetylcholine is not hydrolyzed and its concentration is increased. The resulting accumulation of acetylcholine at the synaptic junctions overstimulates the cholinergic pathways and subsequently desensitizes the cholinergic receptor sites. OP or nerve agents also bind to AChE in the erythrocytes and serum (butyrylcholinesterase

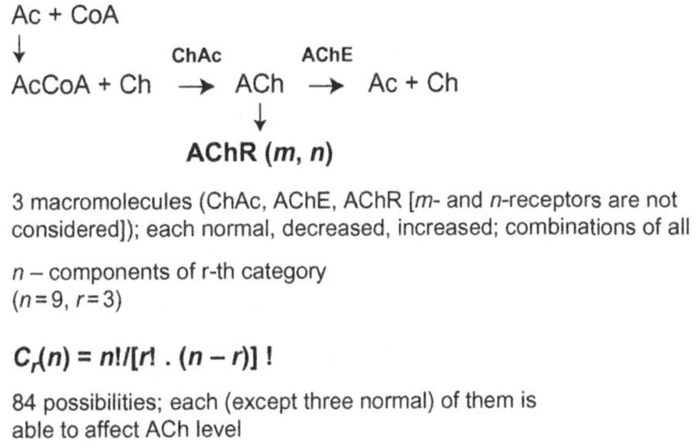

Ac + CoA
↓
AcCoA + Ch —ChAc→ ACh —AChE→ Ac + Ch
↓
AChR (*m*, *n*)

3 macromolecules (ChAc, AChE, AChR [*m*- and *n*-receptors are not considered]); each normal, decreased, increased; combinations of all

n – components of r-th category
($n = 9$, $r = 3$)

$$C_r(n) = n!/[r! \cdot (n - r)]\,!$$

84 possibilities; each (except three normal) of them is able to affect ACh level

Figure 5.1 Three macromolecules involved in cholinergic nerve transmission can be changed and so influence acetylcholine level; possibilities of combinations.

Nerve Agents Poisoning and its Treatment in Schematic Figures and Tables. DOI: 10.1016/B978-0-12-416047-7.00005-0

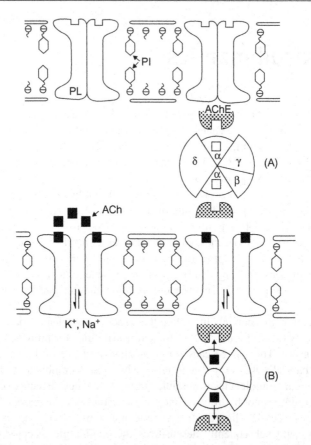

Figure 5.2 Schematic representation of the nicotinic acetylcholine receptor. The proteolipid (PI) receptor is constituting from subunits (α, β, γ, δ); in two subunits, binding sites for acetylcholine are localized (A, cross section). The subunits are forming an ionophore in the membrane, under quiet mode is closed. A nerve impulse (signal) induces neuromediator acetylcholine (ACh) release. The neuromediator is bound to the receptor and changes its conformation: the ionophore is open, and nonequilibrium of ions penetrating through ionophore induces electric potential and the signal is transferred (B, cross section). After signal transmission, ACh is hydrolyzed by AChE, and receptor conformation returns to quiet mode, a new impulse comes, and a new quantum of ACh is released.

BuChE; EC 3.1.1.8); it is pathophysiologically less important, activities of these enzymes (AChE and BuChE) serve as quantitative criterion of exposure.

The differences between these two enzymes (AChE and BuChE) are summarized in Table 5.1. AChE can be characterized as an important enzyme for cholinergic transmission; the function of BuChE is not fully understood. More detailed knowledge of cholinesterases occurred with the description of the molecular structure of AChE. Like other serine hydrolases, AChE contains a catalytic triad called the *esteratic site* (Ser200–His440–Glu327) at the bottom of a deep and narrow cavity known

Effects of organophosphates: inhibition of cholinesterases
(acetylcholinesterase, AChE, EC 3.1.7 and butyrylcholinesterase,
BuChE, EC 3.1.1.8). Other changes (corticosterone, oxygenation, etc.)

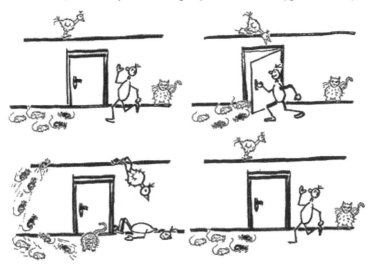

Figure 5.3 Another imagination of the cholinergic nicotinic receptor. Postsynaptic membrane is represented by the wall containing the receptor (door). Released acetylcholine (represented by figure) is bound to the receptor; it changes its conformation, forming an ionophore (open door), and an electric impulse is induced (ions—mice) and the transfer of the impulse is realized. To stop the binding of the neurotransmitter to the receptor, AChE (bird) splits acetylcholine, and the receptor conformation returns to the quiet mode. The next impulse (and acetylcholine) follows, and the action is repeated.

as the *aromatic gorge*. In addition to the catalytic center subsites, AChE possesses one or more additional binding sites for acetylcholine and other quaternary ligands. Such peripheral anionic binding sites are at the lip of this gorge. In BuChE, Trp279, an important component of the peripheral binding site in AChE, is missing. This site is believed to be responsible for substrate inhibition, which is one of the features that distinguishes AChE from BuChE. A hypothetic scheme of the active surface of AChE is given in Figure 5.4.

AChE exists in different molecular forms, some of which seem to be catalytically equivalent. Molecular forms of AChE include globular forms (G) existing as monomers (G1), dimers (G2), and tetramers (G4), preferably in the central nervous system (CNS). These forms are either soluble or membrane associated. The asymmetric forms (A) associated with one, two, or three G forms (A4, A8, A12) are found mainly in peripheral nervous systems and neuromuscular junction.

BuChE is similar to AChE, and there exist a number of genetic variants of this enzyme. The serum–plasma BuChE activity depends on the presence of genetic variants and is lower in comparison with normal genotype. Individuals with lower BuChE activity are more sensitive to cholinesterase inhibitors as well as to drugs

Table 5.1 Differences Between Properties of AChE and BuChE

Trivial Name	Acetylcholinesterase	Butyrylcholinesterase
Other names	Specific, true, "e"-type cholinesterase	Cholinesterase, pseudocholinesterase, "s"-type cholinesterase
Systemic name	Acetylcholine–acetylhydrolase	Acylcholine-acylhydrolase
Number of the enzyme codex	EC 3.1.1.7	EC 3.1.1.8
Main source	Electric organ, brain, erythrocytes	Serum, plasma
Optimal substrate	Acetylcholine	Butyrylcholine
Splitting acetyl-β-methylcholine	Yes	No
Species differences	Low	High
Inhibition by substrate	Yes	No
Quaternary ammonium salts	+++	+
Iso-OMPA	+	+++
Phenothiazines	+++	+
Tacrine	+	+++
DMC	+++	+
Huperzine A	+++	+
Ni, Zn	++	+
Binding	Complex with lipoprotein	Glycoprotein; containing sialic acid
Molecular forms	Subunits	Genetically determined
Molecular weight	69 kDa	85 kDa
Activation Mg, Mn	Mg > Mn	Mg < Mn
Function	Splitting neuromediator acetylcholine	Unknown

Source: Modified from Bajgar (1991, 2004).

split by blood cholinesterases such as succinylcholine or local anesthetics. The AChE forms have different sensitivities to inhibitors as well as to other various factors such as pathological stages, physical factors, and hormones, and this relationship needs to be further studied (for review, see, for example, Bosak et al., 2011; Massoulié et al, 1993; Pohanka, 2011; Wiesner et al., 2007).

The action of OP or nerve agents can be characterized by resorption (penetration into the organism), distribution realized by the transport system (the bloodstream), metabolization, and the toxic effect (AChE inhibition in the central and peripheral nervous systems) (Figure 5.5). However, this scheme can be applicable to all toxic compounds or drugs, adding to the adjective toxic or therapeutic effect.

When these reactions are more specified, it can be demonstrated as shown in Figure 5.6. In this picture, possible materials for laboratory diagnosis are indicated, too. Usually, the blood, erythrocytes, or plasma (serum) are used; in some cases for special diagnosis, other biological fluids are sampled. A more complicated scheme of OP or nerve action is shown in Figure 5.7.

Using a determination of enzyme activity or inhibition in the blood, the effective amount of the nerve agent excluded (because of inhibition) from another toxic

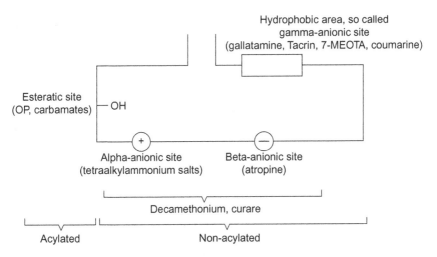

Figure 5.4 Schematic structure of active surface of AChE including different binding sites and differentiation between acylating and nonacylating inhibitors.
Source: Reprinted from Bajgar (2004) with permission.

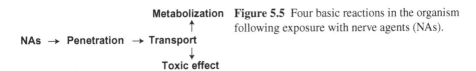

Figure 5.5 Four basic reactions in the organism following exposure with nerve agents (NAs).

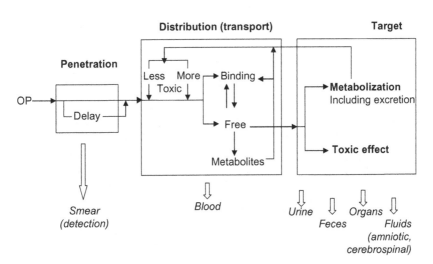

Figure 5.6 Important steps for the action of OPs or nerve agents (**bold**) and possible materials for laboratory diagnosis (*italics*).

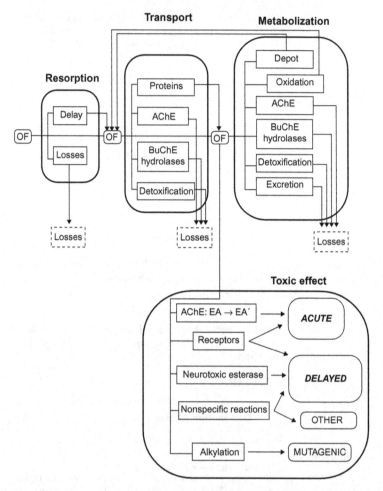

Figure 5.7 A scheme represents four basic actions: absorption, transport, metabolization, and the toxic effect. The absorption is accomplished by OP penetration through biological barriers into the blood representing the transport system. The losses originate either physically or biologically. This part of an OP (reacting by this mechanism) is screened out from toxic action. The losses in the transport system originate from detoxification and nonspecific binding to proteins and enzymes—esterases, AChE, and BuChE. Binding to plasma proteins is also included.
Source: Reprinted from Bajgar (2004) with permission.

action can be assessed—in other words, to assess effective doses especially at different routes of administration (Bajgar and Voicu, 2009). This is logical that following IV administration, the whole dose is acting. Following IM administration, it is a part of the dose administered; the highest losses are observed at PC exposure. It can be pointed out that this calculation involves more inhibiting capacity than the specificity of AChE and BuChE inhibition in the blood (Table 5.2).

Table 5.2 Assessment of Effective Dose of Sarin, Soman, and
VX at Different Routes of Administration in Rats

Route of Administration	Sarin	Soman	VX
IV	93.6	90.1	104.7
IM	55.1	60.3	82.0
IP	20.2	23.2	31.5
PO	5.6	7.1	16.5
PC	0.93	1.2	5.5

Source: Modified from Bajgar (2004); Bajgar and Voicu (2009).

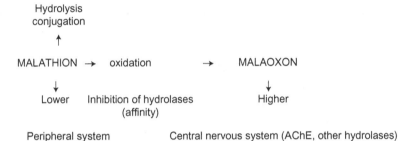

Figure 5.8 Metabolic reactions for malathion. The cytochromes CYP3A4, CYP1A2, and CYP2B6 are involved in the oxidation; however, their role is more complex.

In case of a nonhydrolyzing agent such as VX, IV administration represents the dose inhibiting cholinesterases as such—i.e., inhibition is expected to be 100% (experimental value is about 105%) of the dose administered. In the case of sarin and soman, a part of the administered dose is detoxified, and thus only a portion of the dose administered inhibits blood cholinesterases.

Inhibition of cholinesterases in the blood is practically the first target for an OP or nerve agent, according to the "first come, first served" principle (Benschop and de Jong, 2001). The OP or nerve agent is carried out at the sites of metabolic and toxic effects. However, there are differences especially in the detoxification of highly toxic nerve agents: G agents such as sarin and soman are detoxified, but compounds containing the P-S bond (V agents) are not detoxified (Jokanovic, 2009). On the other hand, thioderivatives are oxidized to oxoderivatives (P=S to P=O; e.g., malathion→malaoxon, parathion→paraoxon). Oxoderivatives can be detoxified, but they are more toxic (lethal synthesis) and stronger cholinesterase inhibitors. Thus, their effects are combination of both reactions, leading to less and more toxic metabolites (Figure 5.8).

The toxic effect site is a multicompartmental system, minimally the central and peripheral nervous systems. In these places, an OP or nerve agent reacts

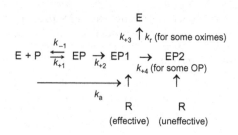

Figure 5.9 Schematic representation of interaction between AChE (E) and an OP (P). The first reaction is forming an intermediate complex (EP) with relevant rate constants (k_{-1}, k_{+1}). A phosphorylated (phosphonylated) enzyme is represented by the first EP complex (EP1) and its rate constant (k_{+2}). This complex (EP1) is able to be reactivated by oximes (reactivators, R)— they are therapeutically effective. The whole reaction is characterized by the bimolecular rate constant of inhibition (k_a), and reactivation is characterized by the rate constant of reactivation (k_{+3}). Depending on the structure of the OP, EP1 can be changed to the second complex EP2 with relevant rate constant (k_{+4}), and this complex is not reactivatable (reactivators are uneffective).

with cholinesterases: AChE and BuChE. Inhibition of cholinesterases is a trigger mechanism for this toxic action. Important nerve agents soman, sarin, and VX are rapidly absorbed at all routes of administration, including inhalation, PC, and oral administration, and they inhibit cholinesterases (preferably AChE) in the central and peripheral nervous systems. Because of soman's high lipophility, it possesses a high affinity to the brain's AChE. Sarin is less lipophilic, however; its affinity to the brain AChE is also very high. Inhibition effects of VX are observed in the periphery, but it is also able to inhibit central AChE.

Thus, cholinesterase inhibition is the basic trigger mechanism of an OP's or a nerve agent's action. Inhibition of cholinesterases, particularly AChE, can be described by simple scheme (Figure 5.9). AChE is represented as the enzyme (E); it is inhibited by OP (P) in two steps to form the intermediate complex enzyme inhibitor (EP). Depending on the structure of the inhibitor, AChE is phosphorylated or phosphonylated; the first complex (EP1) can be reactivated by oximes, whereas complex EP2 is unreactivatable (Figure 5.10).

The principle of this reaction (EP1→EP2; also called *aging*) is releasing the leaving group (alcohol)—i.e., dealkylation (Figure 5.10). Dealkylated (aged) AChE is resistant to oxime's action and to spontaneous reactivation. Therefore, it is one rare example of civilian use of nerve agents: using soman AChE inhibition, the rate of regeneration of AChE can be studied.

Figure 5.11 shows another scheme of inhibition. The scheme for inhibition represents the reactions *in vitro*; it can be applied to the principles of AChE inhibition *in vivo*. It is clear that all these reactions are important for the development of symptoms. The time course of inhibition is important for the sequence of appearance of symptoms; the severity of intoxication depends on the level of the rest of the AChE activity or the level of inhibition, and simultaneously these reactions are important

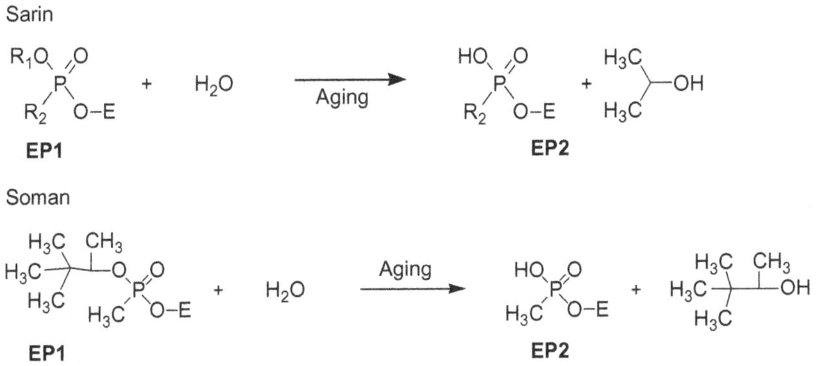

Sarin

Soman

Figure 5.10 The change of reactivatable complex of AChE (E) and OP (EP1) to nonreactivatable complex (EP2) (aging). The molecular mechanism is dealkylation by water forming unreactivatable enzyme and relevant alcohol. Examples for sarin and soman. *Source*: Modified from Bajgar (2004).

for prophylaxis (restoration or protection of AChE against inhibition with nerve agents) and therapeutic countermeasures (the possibility of reactivation).

5.1 Inhibitory Effectiveness

As the basic information (similar to toxicity), anticholinesterase effectivity (affinity) is usually determined. It is characterized by the rate constant k_a (see Figures 5.9 and 5.11) or by the constant I_{50} or IC_{50} (or its negative decadic logarithm—pI_{50}). It is a concentration of inhibitor causing 50% inhibition at given experimental conditions. These two constants are in relationship (equation 5.1):

$$\frac{0.69}{[1]t_{0.5}} = k_a \qquad (5.1)$$

It is difficult to compare the affinities of cholinesterases to nerve agents *in vitro*; there are differences in experimental conditions (source of the enzyme, pH and temperature, time of inhibition, etc.), so the constants pI_{50} demonstrated in Table 5.3 are of an orientation character. However, in general, the affinity of AChE to nerve agents is very high, ranging from 10^{-6} to 10^{-9} M, with corresponding bimolecular rate constants (from 10^5 to 10^8 M/min). Species differences exist but do not vary much among different species, including humans (Table 5.4). In extrapolation experiments, the affinity of nerve agent *in vitro* can be correlated with toxicity *in vivo*. This approach can be applied more easily to highly toxic chemicals such as nerve agents of the V class: the inhibition is very high, and detoxification is low. Moreover, other effects can be limited, too. An example of RVX was given previously (see Figure 4.8).

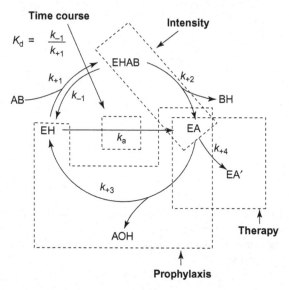

Figure 5.11 In the scheme, EH represents the enzyme (AChE) and AB the inhibitor (nerve agents or OP) with the leaving group B. EHAB is an intermediate complex of AChE and inhibitor and EA phosphorylated enzyme. The complex EA is inactive, and the intensity of poisoning depends on the degree of AChE inhibition. All of these reactions are characterized by the rate constants (k_{+1}, k_{-1}, k_a, k_{+2}, k_{+3}, k_{+4}). The affinity of an enzyme to the inhibitor is expressed as a dissociation constant (K_d). The time course of poisoning depends on the rate of AChE inhibition. OP and nerve agents are potent inhibitors of AChE, having K_d in the range of 10^{-8} to 10^{-9} M. Spontaneous restoration of enzyme activity (EA→EH) is of extremely low rate. It is important for prophylaxis. However, some compounds are able to accelerate the reactivation; called *cholinesterase reactivators*, these drugs are used to treat OP or nerve agent poisoning. Reactivatability also depends on the type of inhibitor. For some nerve agents, it is possible that another reaction called *aging* or *dealkylation* (EA→EA′) involves a chemical reaction in which one of the alkoxyl groups bound to phosphorus is split by water in alcohol form (AOH). This reaction is of great importance for treatment: dealkylated (or aged) AChE is resistant to reactivators. The aging rate is very dependent on the type of nerve agents: the half-life of this dealkylation is the highest for soman-inhibited AChE ($t_{0.5}$—minutes), lower one for sarin ($t_{0.5}$—hours) and for this reaction with VX, the half-life is more than 24 h. This approach can be applied for *in vitro* studies. For *in vivo* action, other specific factors are involved such as distribution of nerve agents into different compartments (thus, their concentrations), penetration of the agent through the blood–brain barrier, and the importance of functional AChE activity in these compartments. When the scheme on inhibition is applied to the principles of AChE inhibition, it is clear that all of these reactions are also important for the development of symptoms (time course and severity of intoxication); simultaneously, these reactions are important for prophylactic and therapeutic countermeasures.

Table 5.3 Affinities of Some Nerve Agents to the Brain AChE

Agent, Source	IC_{50} (M)
VX, rat brain	8.21
VX, human brain	8.1
RVX, rat brain	8.0
RVX, pig brain	8.23
RVX, human brain	8.0
Sarin, rat brain	8.1
GV, rat brain	8.2
Soman, rat brain	8.3
Soman, human brain	8.98
Tabun, rat brain	7.6
Malathion, human brain	4.44

Source: From different sources.

Table 5.4 Bimolecular Rate Constants (k_a) of Interaction of VX to the Brain AChE

Species	$k_a \cdot 10^6$ (M/min)
Humans	1.35
Calf	1.04
Dog	0.91
Rabbit	1.22
Guinea pig	0.68
Rat	1.26
Mouse	0.99

Source: From different sources.

5.2 Other Effects

However, a variety of documented data show that AChE inhibition is not the only important biochemical change during intoxication. Many other changes accompanied with the development of intoxication that might contribute to OP toxicity have been described. They include changes of other enzymes, neurotransmitters, immune changes, anaphylactoid reaction, and behavior, among others. The evidence includes the data indicating that prophylactics or therapeutic drugs might also have multiple sites of action similar to those observed during intoxication.

Schematic representation of OP or nerve agent action on different systems is shown in Figure 5.12.

The delayed neurotoxic effect is caused by a reason different from cholinesterase inhibition. The neurotoxic esterase has been described as the target site for this

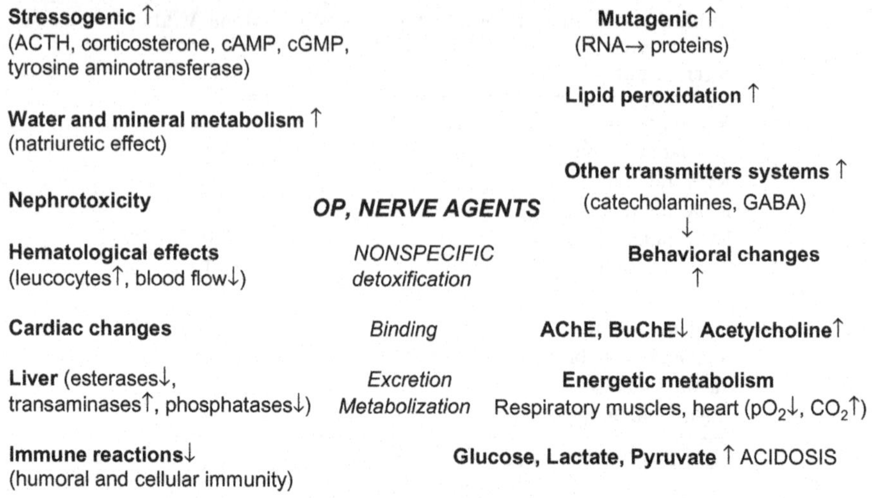

Stressogenic ↑
(ACTH, corticosterone, cAMP, cGMP,
tyrosine aminotransferase)

Water and mineral metabolism ↑
(natriuretic effect)

Nephrotoxicity

Hematological effects
(leucocytes↑, blood flow↓)

Cardiac changes

Liver (esterases↓,
transaminases↑, phosphatases↓)

Immune reactions↓
(humoral and cellular immunity)

OP, NERVE AGENTS

NONSPECIFIC
detoxification

Binding

Excretion
Metabolization

Mutagenic ↑
(RNA→ proteins)

Lipid peroxidation ↑

Other transmitters systems ↑
(catecholamines, GABA)
↓
Behavioral changes
↑

AChE, BuChE↓ Acetylcholine↑

Energetic metabolism
Respiratory muscles, heart (pO_2↓, CO_2↑)

Glucose, Lactate, Pyruvate ↑ ACIDOSIS

Figure 5.12 Schematic representation of some reactions accompanied with OP nerve agent actions. They are complex changes of very different character.
Source: Modified from Allon et al. (2007); Bloch-Shilderman and Levy (2007); Bajgar (2004); Marrs et al. (1996); and Gupta (2009).

symptom; however, only some OPs are neurotoxic in that sense. A typical example is tri-*o*-cresyl phosphate.

Another action of nerve agents is observed in a relatively long time interval (weeks) after the exposure (Kassa et al., 2007). It can be characterized by behavioral changes determined using the Functional Observation Battery. In Table 5.5, all observed parameters are summarized, and Tables 5.6 and 5.7 show the results following inhalation exposure of guinea pigs to soman vapors 1 day and 4 weeks after the exposure. These changes cannot be fully explained by AChE inhibition, and they result from an imbalance of neurotransmitters. Although these findings are difficult to extrapolate directly to human low-level exposures to OPs or nerve agents, they indicate that the previously mentioned alteration of various physiological functions—including subtle neurophysiological and behavioral dysfunctions, and spatial discrimination impairments without clinically manifested disturbance of the central cholinergic nervous system—could also occur in humans for a relatively long time (from weeks to months) following the inhalation exposure to asymptomatic or nonconvulsive symptomatic levels of nerve agents (see also Bajgar, 2009; Gupta, 2009).

During the acute phase of OP or nerve agent poisoning, the accumulation of acetylcholine induces clinical symptoms of acute poisoning. They are similar for nerve agents and OP, although the time of symptoms is different (Figure 5.13). For differential diagnosis, Table 5.8 summarizes the time sequelae of symptoms during intoxication with different CWA. The assessed toxicity of selected nerve agents for humans is given in Table 5.9.

Table 5.5 List of Behavioral Characteristics and Scores Given According to the Extent of Severity of the Symptoms Observed

Characteristics	Severity of Symptoms and Corresponding Scores									
	-2	-1	0	1	2	3	4	5	6	7
Posture				Sitting or standing	Rearing	Asleep	Flattened	Lying on side	Crouched over	Head bobbing
Catch difficulty				Passive	Normal	Defense	Flight	Escape	Aggression	
Ease of handling				Very easy	Normal	Moderately difficult	Difficult			
Muscular tonus	Atonia	Hypotonia	Normal	Hypertonia	Rigidity					
Lacrimation			None	Slight	Severe	Crusta	Colored crusta			
Palpebral closure				Open	Slightly drooping	Halfway drooping	Completely shut	Ptosis		
Endo- or exophthalmus		Endo	Normal	Exo						
Fur abnormalities			None	Colored	Tousled	Colored + tousled	Blaze	Injury	Other changes	Pilo-erection
Skin abnormalities			Normal	Pale	Erythema	Cyanosis	Pigmented	Cold	Injury	
Salivation			None	Slight	Severe					
Nose secretion			None	Slight	Severe	Colored				
Clonic movements			Normal	Repetitive movements of mouth and jaws	Nonrhythmic quivers	Mild tremors	Severe tremors	Myoclonic jerks	Clonic convulsions	
Tonic movements			Normal	Contraction of extensors	Opisthotonus	Emprosthotonus	Explosive jumps	Tonic convulsions		

(Continued)

Table 5.5 (Continued)

Characteristics	-2	-1	0	1	2	3	4	5	6	7
Gait			*Normal*	Ataxia	Overcompensation of hind limb movements	Feet point outward from body	Forelimbs are extended	Walks on tiptoes	Hunched body	Body is flattened against surface
Gait score				*Normal*	Slightly impaired	Somewhat impaired	Totally impaired			
Mobility score				*Normal*	Slightly impaired	Somewhat impaired	Totally impaired			
Arousal[a]				Very low	Sporadic	Reduced	*Normal*	Enhanced		
Tension			None	Partial (ears)	Stupor					
Vocalism			None	Induced	Spontaneous	Excessive				
Stereotypy			None	Head weaving	Body weaving	Grooming	Circling	Others	Permanent	
Bizarre behavior			None	Head	Body	Self-mutilation	Abnormal movements	Others		
Approach response				No reaction	*Normal*	Freeze	Energetic reaction	Exaggerated reaction		
Touch response				No reaction	*Normal*	Freeze	Energetic reaction	Exaggerated reaction		
Click response				No reaction	*Normal*	Freeze	Energetic reaction	Exaggerated reaction		

Parameter							
Tail-pinch response	No reaction	*Normal*	Freeze	Energetic reaction	Exaggerated reaction		
Pupil size	Miosis considerable	Miosis slight	*Normal*	Mydriasis slight	Mydriasis considerable		
Pupil response	No reaction	*Normal reaction*					
Righting reflex	*Normal*	Slightly uncoordinated	Lands on side	Lands on back	Rise from back spontaneously	Rise from back with stimulus	No reaction
Landing foot splay (mm)	Measured in mm						
Food receiving (%)	Measured in percentage with respect to control animals						
Vertical activity	Number of activities per 10min						
Horizontal activity	Number of activities per 10min						
Total motor activity	Number of activities per 10min						

Table 5.6 Behavioral Characteristics Out of a Total Number of 36 That Are Significantly Affected by Inhalatory Exposure of Guinea Pigs to At Least One of Three Concentrations of Soman Vapor in Air for 60 min as Observed 1 Day After Exposure

Characteristics	Scores[a] Given After Exposure to a Soman Concentration[b]			
	0 mg/m^3	1.2 mg/m^3	1.5 mg/m^3	2.7 mg/m^3
Ease of handling	2 ± 0	2 ± 0	2 ± 0	$1.5 \pm 0.6^*$
Tonic movements	0 ± 0	$0.5 \pm 0.6^*$	$0.5 \pm 0.6^*$	$0.8 \pm 0.4^{**}$
Gait	0 ± 0	0.8 ± 2.0	$1.2 \pm 1.2^*$	$0.8 \pm 0.4^{**}$
Gait score	1 ± 0	$1.5 \pm 0.6^*$	$1.8 \pm 0.4^{**}$	$2.0 \pm 0^{**}$
Mobility score	1 ± 0	1 ± 0	1.3 ± 0.5	$1.7 \pm 0.5^*$
Arousal	4 ± 0	4.2 ± 0.4	3.5 ± 1.1	$4.7 \pm 0.5^*$
Vocalism	1.7 ± 0.8	2 ± 1	1.2 ± 1.3	$2.7 \pm 0.5^*$
Approach response	2 ± 0	$2.5 \pm 0.6^*$	2.5 ± 0.8	$3.0 \pm 0.9^*$
Touch response	2 ± 0	2.3 ± 0.8	2 ± 0	$3.0 \pm 0.9^*$
Click response	2 ± 0	2 ± 0	2 ± 0	$3.3 \pm 1.0^*$
Pupil size	0 ± 0	$-1.0 \pm 0^{**}$	$-0.8 \pm 0.4^{**}$	-0.3 ± 0.5

Scores for the extent of severity of the symptoms are given as well as values for untreated animals.
[a]Mean values ($n = 6$) $\pm$ SD; $^*0.01 < P < 0.05$, $^{**}P < 0.001$.
[b]The three doses correspond to 0.3, 0.4, and 0.7 LCt$_{50}$.
Source: Modified from Bajgar et al. (2004b).

Table 5.7 Behavioral Characteristics Out of a Total Number of 36 That Are Significantly Affected by Inhalatory Exposure of Guinea Pigs to At Least One of Three Concentrations of Soman Vapor in Air for 60 min as Observed 4 Weeks After Exposure

Characteristics	Scores[a] Given After Exposure to a Soman Concentration[b]			
	0 mg/m^3	1.2 mg/m^3	1.5 mg/m^3	2.7 mg/m^3
Catch difficulty	3.8 ± 0.5	2.7 ± 0.5	$2.5 \pm 0.8^*$	3.3 ± 0.5
Ease of handling	2.8 ± 0.5	2.5 ± 0.6	2.5 ± 0.8	$1.3 \pm 0.8^*$
Muscular tonus	0 ± 0	0 ± 0	0.3 ± 0.5	$0.5 \pm 0.6^*$
Vocalism	1.8 ± 0.5	1.0 ± 1.1	$0.5 \pm 0.8^*$	$0.5 \pm 0.8^*$
Approach response	2 ± 0	2.2 ± 0.4	2.5 ± 0.8	$3.3 \pm 1.0^*$
Touch response	2 ± 0	2 ± 0	2 ± 0	$3.2 \pm 0.8^*$
Click response	2 ± 0	2 ± 0	2 ± 0	$3.0 \pm 0.9^*$
Horizontal activity	52 ± 44	61 ± 33	75 ± 65	$160 \pm 23^*$
Total motor activity	54 ± 46	62 ± 33	76 ± 65	$170 \pm 29^*$

[a]Mean values ($n = 6$) $\pm$ SD; $^*0.01 < P < 0.05$.
[b]The three doses correspond to 0.3, 0.4, and 0.7 LCt$_{50}$.
Source: Modified from Bajgar et al. (2004b).

Nerve agents (min)	CENTRAL	OP (h)
(0–30)	Giddiness, anxiety, restlessness, *headache*, tremor, *confusion*, failure to concentration, convulsions *disturbed breathing*, respiratory depression	(0.5–2)

	MUSCARINIC	
0–5	Increased secretion — rhinorrhea, *salivation*,	0–1
5–10	lacrimation, *bronchorrhea*, sweating,	1–3
10–15	*miosis*, failure of accomodation, abdominal cramp, diarrhea, bradycardia, hypotension, involuntary micturition	3–8

	NICOTINIC	
20–60	*Weakness, fasciculations, convulsions*, generalized convulsions	2–8

	DEATH	
30–60	Failure of heart and ventilation functions	2–24

The most typical symptoms are in italics bold

Figure 5.13 Symptoms of intoxication with OPs and nerve agents.
Source: Modified from Bajgar (2004); Marrs et al. (1996).

5.3   Cholinesterase Determination

Diagnosis of intoxication is based on the observation of clinical symptoms and laboratory examination. Materials for clinical laboratory were briefly mentioned in Figure 5.6. The most accessible is the blood. The possibilities for laboratory testing are shown in Figure 5.14.

The determination of cholinesterases in the blood is the basic method for diagnosis and therapy monitoring for OP poisoning, though some doubts exist preferring the clinical signs of poisoning as a leading tool for OP poisoning diagnosis and monitoring. The determination of AChE and BuChE activity in the whole blood is possible.

Determination of cholinesterase activity is based on many principles. In general, an enzyme is added to the buffered mixture, and the enzymatic reaction is initiated by adding the substrate. Different parts of the reaction mixture are determined (continually or discontinually)—i.e., unhydrolyzed substrate or reaction products, either directly or indirectly (Figure 5.15).

According to the procedure and laboratory instrumentation, the most common methods of cholinesterase determination are as follows: electrometrical, titration, manometric, colorimetric detection of the unhydrolyzed substrate, measurement by

Table 5.8 Important Poisoning Symptoms of Different Types of CWAs and Time (min) of Their Appearance

Agent	0–10	10–30	30–60	60–120	120–480
Nerve agents	Giddiness, anxiety, restlessness, headache, breathing difficulties, miosis	Confusion, salivation, lacrimation, bronchorrhea, sweating, respiratory depression, tremor	Weakness, fasciculations, convulsions	Generalized convulsions, metabolic disbalance, paralysis of heart and ventilation	Death
Blistering agents	No	No	Nausea (vomiting), eye smarting	Erythema, vertigo, skin stretching, pain, slight edema, bronchosecretion	Development of vesicles (24–48 h), bronchopneumonia; later (days to weeks) immunity decrease
Cyanides	Smelling of bitter almonds, hyperventilation, anxiety	Unconsciousness, mydriasis, convulsions	Convulsions and death		
Irritants	Sneezing, cough, lacrimation, pain, eye irritation	Persistent difficulties mentioned, respiratory tract irritation, nausea			
Asphyxiating	No	No substantial breathing difficulties, bronchorrhea, tightness in the chest	Without substantial symptoms	Latency	Dyspnea, lung edema development
Incapacitants	No	Dry mouth, mucosas, mydriasis, rubego		Confusion, anxiety	Development of all types of hallucinations, long lasting (hours), lethargy later on (24 h), amnesia

Table 5.9 Assessed Toxicity of Nerve Agents for Humans

Agent	Inhalation Toxicity, LCT_{50} (mg/min/m^3)	PC toxicity, LD_{50} (mg/70 kg)
Sarin	150–400	500–2,000
Soman	70–200	500–1,500
VX	15–60	10–50
Tabun	400–600	500–2,000
Cyclosarin	500–700	30–80
GV	20–70	50–100

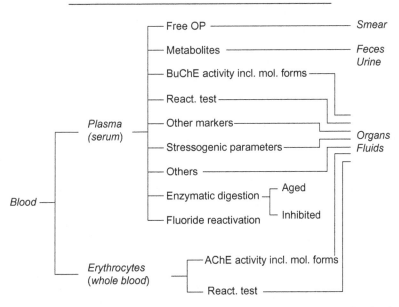

Figure 5.14 Possible methods for laboratory diagnosis of OP or nerve agent poisoning in the blood.

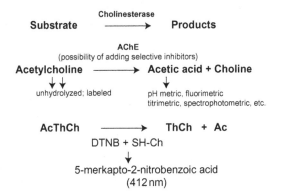

Figure 5.15 Principles and methods for cholinesterase determination.

the change of pH using an indicator, spectrophotometric, fluorimetric, radiometric, calorimetric, polarographic, enzymatic, and others (e.g., near-infrared spectroscopy). These methods are also suitable for the detection of cholinesterase inhibitors using biosensors or immunochemical assay for detection of CWA.

A very sensitive and commonly used method for cholinesterase determination was described by Ellman et al. (1961), based on hydrolysis of the thiocholine substrates (acetyl- and butyrylthiocholine or others). After enzymatic hydrolysis, the relevant acid and thiocholine are released, and thiocholine is detected by its SH-group using 5,5'dithiobis-2 nitrobenzoic acid as it forms 5-mercapto-2-nitrobenzoate anion determined spectrophotometrically at 412 nm. Sometimes this method is used with specific inhibitors, and there are many modifications described in the literature. This method is in good correlation with other methods. It is sufficiently specific and sensitive, and it is used for different purposes in many laboratories around the world. An expression of the activity varies greatly, usually as μmoles of substrate hydrolyzed per min (time) per ml of the examined material (e.g., plasma, serum) or per mg of weight tissue (wet, dry, mg of nitrogen, etc.). From these values, the expression of the activity in units can be derived (it is the quantity of enzyme catalyzing μmol of substrate per min at standard conditions). In the clinical laboratory, the activity can be also expressed as catal per liter—i.e., 1 mol of substrate hydrolyzed per sec per liter or kg (cat/l, kg), which is the hydrolysis of 1 mol of substrate hydrolyzed per sec per liter or kg.

An interesting modification for determining AChE activity is the use of quantitative histochemistry: in studies dealing with the mechanism of nerve agents action *in vivo*, AChE inhibition or reactivation in different tissues as a marker of the effect is determined. Homogenates of different tissues are used for biochemical AChE determination, not allowing changes in different structures including the brain and its areas to be detected. The quantitative histochemical determination of AChE activity allows fine differentiation for various brain structures and quantifies these changes (Figure 5.16). Though AChE inhibition detected biochemically showed a similar degree of inhibition, the quantitative histochemistry of AChE demonstrated that inhibition effects are different for various inhibitors. The results showed that AChE activity or inhibition detected by quantitative histochemistry is more informative than the determination of AChE activity or inhibition in homogenates of the brain parts using biochemical methods. Moreover, the results of both methods (histo- and biochemical) correlate very well (Bajgar et al., 2007). The brain is a complex organ containing different AChE activities in its structure (Gupta, 2004). There are 10-fold differences between, for example, the striatum and the cerebellum. When the activity is determined in the whole brain homogenate, the final result is a "mean" activity, though the activities in different areas are different. A similar situation can be observed in any case in which the sample is not enzymatically homogenous: it contains either different enzymes (blood, erythrocyte AChE, and plasma BuChE) and it differs in their activities (brain parts, also the content of AChE and BuChE) or in the content of molecular AChE forms having different activities.

Many publications deal with the review and modifications of cholinesterase determination. A continual determination of the rat blood cholinesterase activity (Bajgar, 1991; new modification Cabal et al., 2010) is interesting and useful.

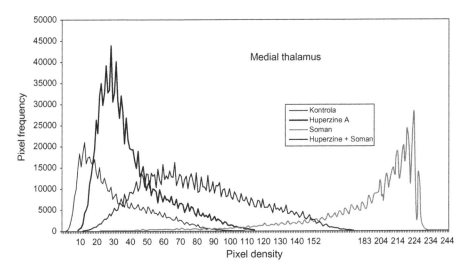

Figure 5.16 Quantitative histochemistry of AChE detection in the medial thalamus of the rat brain. The effects of soman and Huperzine A in comparison with control. Methodical details were described previously (Bajgar et al., 2007). Quantitative evaluation was kindly submitted by Dr. P. Hajek, Department of Anatomy, Medical Faculty, Charles University in Hradec Kralove.

Using this continual monitoring, it is possible to differentiate changes in blood cholinesterase activity following different experimental conditions—e.g., in various routes of administration, in monitoring a reactivator's effect, and other modifications of blood enzyme after being influenced by different factors (Figure 5.17). An original record is given in Figure 5.18. Currently, the activity is represented by the whole blood cholinesterases, although differentiating between erythrocyte AChE and plasma BuChE would be possible.

The decrease in these activities is a good marker, but the diagnostic validity is limited to the statement that some factors causing a decrease in blood cholinesterases are present. In connection with the anamnestic data (exposure to OP), this is important information. The determination of the red blood cell AChE or plasma BuChE is more informative. AChE activity in the red blood cell can be considered more important for diagnosis with the nerve agents than the plasma BuChE activity. For acute intoxication with nerve agents, the correlation between clinical signs of poisoning and red blood cells AChE activity was demonstrated (Figure 5.19). For later stages of intoxication, AChE activity remains decreased but without marked clinical symptoms.

For occupational medicine purposes, the determination of cholinesterases in the blood of workers with OP is obligatory. A decrease of the activity below 70% of normal values is an indicator that the worker should not come into contact with OP. However, the normal values varied within the laboratories, depending on the method of determination. According to our experience, the determination of individual

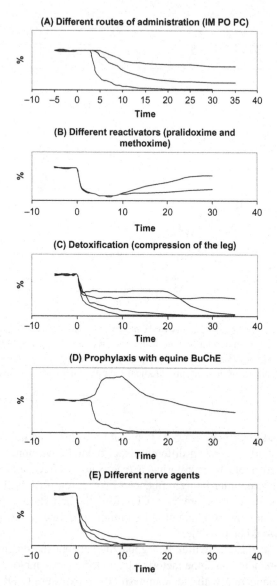

(A) Different routes of administration (IM PO PC)

(B) Different reactivators (pralidoxime and methoxime)

(C) Detoxification (compression of the leg)

(D) Prophylaxis with equine BuChE

(E) Different nerve agents

Figure 5.17 Examples of the use of continual determination of rat blood cholinesterase activity *in vivo*. Simplified (and redrafted into one picture) curves of enzyme determination are shown. For illustration, the original follows (Figure 5.18). (A) Changes in the blood cholinesterase activity following IM (left), PO (middle), and PC (right) administration of sarin. (B) Changes in the blood cholinesterase activity following intoxication with sarin treated with atropine and methoxime (up) or pralidoxime (bottom). (C) Changes in the blood cholinesterase activity following intoxication (IM administration into the leg) with sarin and VX. One minute later, the leg was compressed; 20 min later, compression was released. Thin line = sarin; thick line = VX. Following relaxation, inhibition with VX continues; inhibition with sarin is not observed—the toxic agent was detoxified. (D) Changes in the blood cholinesterase activity following prophylaxis with equine BuChE; activity is increased. Following sarin administration (10 min), activity is recorded. Bottom is the record of pretreatment with saline only. (E) Changes in the blood cholinesterase activity following IM administration of soman (left), sarin (middle), and VX (right).

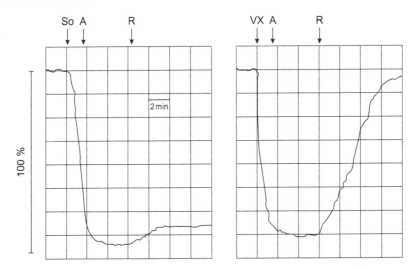

Figure 5.18 Original records (copies) of cholinesterase determination in rat blood. Left: IM administration of soman (arrow) and treatment with atropine (A) and methoxime (R). Right: Inhibition with VX, atropine, and methoxime. Note that administration of atropine did not change the blood cholinesterase activity. After administration of reactivator, small reactivation in case of soman was observed (later on, aging probably occurs); in case of VX, full reactivation was demonstrated.

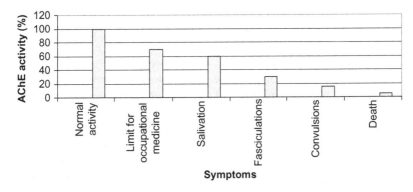

Figure 5.19 AChE activity in erythrocytes and symptoms of poisoning following acute exposure to nerve agents.

cholinesterase (or AChE and BuChE) normal activity before contact or work with OPs or nerve agents is optimal.

The direct determinations of the toxic agent (OP or a nerve agent) in the circulating system are also possible. However, the parent compound will circulate intact for a short period of time, and detection will not be possible for more than approximately hours after exposure. Metabolites circulate for a longer period of time and are mostly excreted in urine. A metabolite of sarin (O-isopropyl methylphosphonic acid) could be traced in urine and plasma from victims after the Tokyo subway sarin terrorist attack. For some OP pesticides (parathion, paraoxon), the detection of p-nitrophenol in urine is an indicator of exposure. However, the retrospectivity of these methods is limited. The detection using an immunoassay of nerve agents is in progress. The antibodies against soman may have the appropriate specificity and affinity for immunodiagnosis of soman exposure.

The methods for determining blood cholinesterases' inhibition (AChE and BuChE) do not allow identification of the OP and do not provide reliable evidence for exposure at inhibition levels less than 10–20%. Moreover, they are less suitable for retrospective detection of exposure because of de novo synthesis of enzymes. A relatively new method was developed that is based on reactivation of phosphylated cholinesterase and carboxylesterase (CaE) by fluoride ions. Treatment of the inhibited enzyme with fluoride ions can inverse the inhibition reaction yielding a restored enzyme and a phosphofluoridate that is subsequently isolated and quantified by gas chromatography and phosphorus-specific or mass spectrometric detection. Human (and monkey) plasma does not contain CaE, but its BuChE concentration is relatively high (70–80 nM), much higher than the concentration of AChE in blood (cca 3 nM). The plasma of laboratory animals such as rats and guinea pigs contains considerable concentrations of CaE in addition to cholinesterases. This method allows a partial identification of the OP, whereas the lifetime of the phosphylated esterase (and consequently the retrospectivity of the method) is only limited by spontaneous reactivation, in vivo sequestration, and aging. The rate of the latter process (aging) depends on the structure of the phosphyl moiety bound to the enzyme and on the type of esterase. Phosphylated CaEs generally do not age. Based on this method for retrospective detection of exposure to OP, the exposure of victims of the Tokyo incident to an OP, probably sarin, could be established from analysis of their blood samples. Fluoride-induced reactivation of OP-inhibited AChE is a reliable and retrospective method to establish OP exposure. It is limited to compounds that regenerate with fluoride ions. Another procedure for diagnosis of exposure to OP that surpasses the limitations of the fluoride reactivation method was described. It is based on the rapid isolation of BuChE from the plasma by the affinity chromatography, digestion with pepsin, followed by liquid chromatography, with the mass spectrometric analysis of phosphylated nonapeptides resulting after the digestion of inhibited BuChE with pepsin. The method can be applied for the detection of exposures to various OP pesticides and nerve agents, including soman. This approach is very valuable and represents a new field for the improvement of diagnosis with nerve agents and OP (for review, see, for example, Bajgar, 2005; Fidder et al., 2002; Noort et al., 2009).

As previously mentioned, a decrease in cholinesterase activity is the factor indicating (after the exclusion of other factors) an exposure to OPs or nerve agents or other cholinesterase inhibitors. This simple determination does not allow us to make some decisions dealing with the antidotal therapy (especially the repeated administration of reactivators), and then it has a low prognostic validity. Therefore, a new test of the reactivation has been described. The principle of the reactivation test is double determination of the enzyme, the first without and the second one with the presence

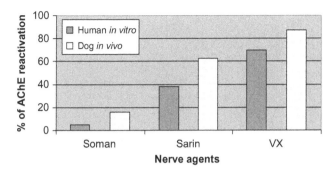

Figure 5.20 Reactivation (%) of the human blood AChE *in vitro* and the dog blood AChE *in vivo* following sarin, soman, and VX exposure.

of a reactivator in the sample. The choice of reactivator depends on the availability of the oxime, although in principle it is necessary to have the same concentrations of the reagents in these parallel samples. The concentration of the reactivator (usually trimedoxime, but other oximes such as obidoxime, pralidoxime, or HI-6 are also possible) must not be higher than the oxime concentration that causes the hydrolysis of the substrate (acetyl- or butyrylthiocholine)—i.e., the oxime concentration is lower than 10^{-3} M because these higher concentrations of oximes cause artificial hydrolysis of the substrate. Using this method, *in vitro* reactivation of the whole human blood *in vitro* inhibited by various nerve agents (VX, sarin, soman) was determined. This reactivation test was used to determine the reactivatability in rats and dogs intoxicated with the same nerve agents (sarin, soman, and VX). The results of the reactivation *in vivo* in dogs and *in vitro* in human are shown in Figure 5.20. From these results, differential diagnosis can be derived—in the case of low reactivation (0–10%), soman as the toxic agent is the most probable. A middle reactivation of about 50% indicates sarin intoxication, and a high reactivation is typical for VX. In this connection, a portable, rapid, and sensitive assessment of subclinical OP exposure based on reactivation of OP-inhibited cholinesterase using rat saliva *in vitro* was developed using an electrochemical sensor coupled with a microflow-injection system (Du et al., 2009).

The gene-expression profile after nerve agent intoxication was also studied (Gopalakrishnakone, 2003; Sprading et al., 2011), and in the future these results can be an important contribution to our knowledge of the mechanism of action as well as to new approaches to antidotal treatment.

Conclusions

The pharmacodynamics of nerve agent action is basically known: it is triggered by AChE inhibition and is followed by other changes, although it contains some gaps. A solution of these previously unclear questions will not only contribute to better understanding of the pathogenesis of nerve agent action but also will contribute to our knowledge in pharmacology and neuropharmacology in general.

6 Antidotal Treatment

Based on our knowledge of the mechanism of action, the following therapeutic countermeasures for antidotal treatment are used. The main drugs are anticholinergics (preferably atropine); their formulas and dosing are shown in Figures 6.1 and 6.2; reactivators and anticonvulsants are other current antidotes.

Anticholinergics antagonize the effects of accumulated acetylcholine at the cholinergic synapses (also called *symptomatic antidotes*) and cholinesterase reactivators (oximes) reactivate inhibited AChE (*causal antidotes*). Their effects are synergistic. Benzodiazepines are also used to treat convulsions (anticonvulsants, usually diazepam). Treatment of metabolic dysbalance, ionic hypoequilibrium, and support of vital functions (heart, ventilation) is necessary. The use of atropine is without any discussion; other anticholinergics may be even more efficacious. The centrally acting anticholinergics (benactyzine, biperidene) can be very useful in the therapy of soman poisoning. Anticonvulsants (diazepam) in the treatment of OP or nerve agent poisoning are also frequently used. However, the use of reactivators is a more complicated question (Figure 6.3).

General treatment is based on regulation of homeostasis, especially oxygenation and stability of the blood pH. Many factors impair this situation (Figure 6.4).

The choice of reactivators is not so simple. Their administration alone is not effective, but simultaneous administration with atropine potentiates their antidotal effects based on AChE reactivation at the cholinergic nerve synapses. AChE reactivation at the peripheral nervous system is indisputable; however, as demonstrated, passing through the blood–brain barrier facilitating its central reactivation efficacy *in vivo*. Though the research is

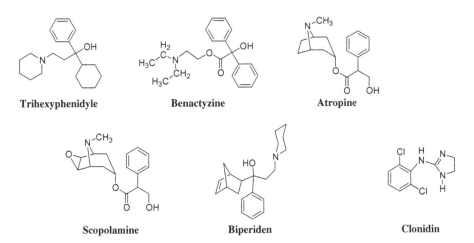

Figure 6.1 Chemical formulas of some anticholinergics.

Nerve Agents Poisoning and its Treatment in Schematic Figures and Tables. DOI: 10.1016/B978-0-12-416047-7.00006-2

- Atropine   2–5 mg IV, IM
- Benactyzine   1–2 mg PO
- Scopolamine   0.5–1.0 mg IV, IM
- Trasentine   50–100 mg IM
- Tiphen   20–30 mg PO
- Tropacine   10–12.5 mg PO
- Parpanite   25–100 mg PO
- Biperidene   2–4 mg PO
- Trihexyphenidyle 1–2 mg PO

Figure 6.2 Recommended doses of anticholinergics for the treatment of OP or nerve agent intoxication.

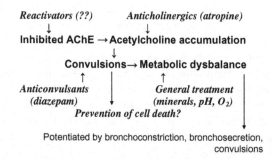

Figure 6.3 Simple scheme of action of organophosphorus cholinesterase inhibitors: inhibition of AChE causes accumulation of neuromediator acetylcholine followed by convulsions and metabolic disbalance (changes in the mineral concentration, blood and tissue pH, and oxygen saturation). Possible therapeutic countermeasures are given in *italics*. When the choice of anticholinergics and anticonvulsives is more clear, the choice of reactivators remains an open question. An interesting approach was described by Collombet (2011): for the first time, brain cell therapy and neuronal regeneration were considered as a valuable contribution toward delayed treatment against OP or nerve agent intoxication. Similarly, prevention or treatment of neuronal death is another problem.
Source: Modified from Bajgar (2004), Gupta (2009), and Patocka (2004).

very intensive, unfortunately, until now there has not been a universal or significantly better reactivator that is sufficiently effective against all nerve agents or OPs when compared with currently available oximes. As described many times, only a few commercially available AChE reactivators are on the market: pralidoxime (2-PAM; P2S; 2-hydroxy-iminomethyl-1-methylpyridinium chloride or methansulphonate), trimedoxime [Fosan®, 1,3-bis(4-hydroxyiminomethylpyridinium)-propane dichloride or dibromide], obidox-ime [Toxogonin®; LüH-6; 1,3-bis(4-hydroxyiminomethylpyridinium)-2-oxapropane dichloride], methoxime [MMC-4; MMB-4; 1,1-bis(4-hydroxyiminomethylpyridinium)-methane dichloride or dibromide] and HI-6 [1-(2-hydroxyiminomethylpyridinium)-3-(4-carbamoylpyridinium)–2-oxapropane dichloride or dimethanesulfonate] (Figure 6.5).

The toxicity of reactivators is variable (Table 6.1); there are no considerable sex differences—e.g., IM toxicity of HI-6 is 639.7 mg/kg for female rats and 779.7 for male rats. The same values for mice are 638.8 (female) and 662.4 (male) mg/kg,

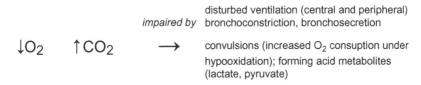

$$\downarrow O_2 \qquad \uparrow CO_2 \qquad \longrightarrow$$

impaired by

disturbed ventilation (central and peripheral) bronchoconstriction, bronchosecretion

convulsions (increased O_2 consuption under hypooxidation); forming acid metabolites (lactate, pyruvate)

Figure 6.4 Different factors involved in development of O_2 and CO_2 blood saturation following nerve agent or OP poisoning.

respectively. Recommended doses of reactivators available for human use are given in Figure 6.6.

There were synthesized many new oximes; unfortunately, none is able to reactivate AChE inhibited by all nerve agents and OP pesticides. Some new oximes were shown in Figure 6.5; some of them are under research because of their good reactivatability for AChE inhibited by OP pesticides (K 048) or by tabun (K 203). However, because of fast dealkylation of AChE inhibited by soman (aging), treatment of soman intoxication using reactivators seems to be a special problem (Voicu et al., 2010). The choice of antidotes is relatively large. Used drugs were demonstrated in Figure 6.5; for human use, smaller number of oximes is available (Figure 6.6). However, AChE reactivation is not the only reaction of reactivators (Figure 6.7). They are also able to inhibit AChE (at higher concentrations) to influence acetylcholine metabolism (high-affinity choline uptake), and they have anticholinergic properties varying from one oxime to another (Soukup et al., 2010); it is probably a reason for their therapeutic effect without AChE reactivation. Another problem is their relative hepatotoxicity observed in some reactivators (e.g., trimedoxime), which limits their human use.

6.1 Therapeutic and Reactivation Effectiveness

Therapeutic efficacy can be tested by many methods. The most obvious is determination of therapeutic (protective) index—i.e., the ratio of the LD_{50} of treated animals to the LD_{50} of untreated animals. Another possibility is the method of isoboles (Figure 6.8). It can be used for more precise determination of therapeutic interaction such as synergistic or summation effects, but this method is expensive and requires a large amount of experimental animals.

Reactivation *in vitro* can be monitored using a kinetic approach: the kinetics of reactivation is represented by the reaction

$$EI + R \xrightarrow{K_R} EIR \xrightarrow{k_R} E + P$$

where EI is OP (or nerve agent)-inhibited enzyme; R is the reactivator; E is the reactivated enzyme; EIR is the intermediate complex; P is the product, usually phosphorylated oxime (unstable); and K_R and k_R are the relevant dissociation and rate constants for decomposition of the intermediate complex, respectively. Thus, K_R

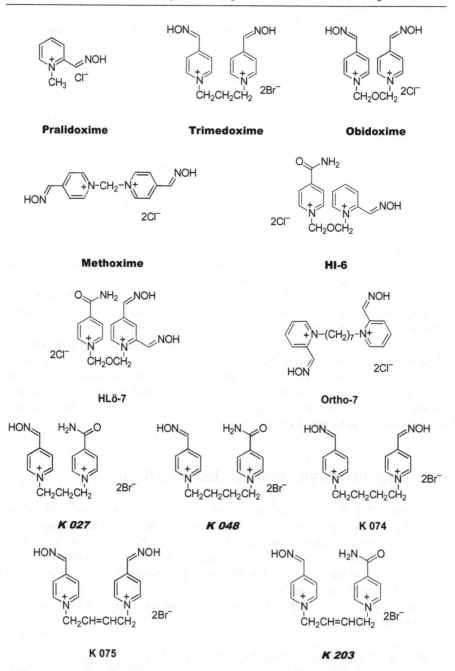

Figure 6.5 Structures of some reactivators. Clinically important oximes are in bold; prospective reactivators are in bold italics; they are K 048 and K 027 (prospective against organophosphorus insecticides) and K 203 (against tabun).

Table 6.1 Toxicities of Different Reactivators

Reactivator	Toxicity, IM (LD$_{50}$, mg/kg)		
	Rats	Mice	Mice IP
Trimedoxime	150.5	149.3	73.5
Obidoxime	211.1 (158.4)	188.4	–
Pralidoxime	218.0	263.6	–
Methoxime	641.8	441.4	–
HI-6	781.3	671.3	448.4
HLö-7	564.1	543.2	–
K 027	>1,200	–	672.8
K 048	>1,200	233.5	224.9
K 074	49.0	–	21.4
K 075	71.3	–	–
K 203	326.4	95.0	–
K 156	127.4	84.0	–
K 250	>800	555.6	–
K 251	358.2	116.1	–
K 033	–	47.9	–

Toxicity of HI-6 (IM): LD$_{50}$, guinea pig 500 mg/kg; dog 350 mg/kg.
Source: According to Bartosova et al. (2006); Kuca et al. (2011); Kuca and Kassa (2003).

- Pralidoxime iodide   0.5–1.0 g IV, IM
- Pralidoxime chloride   0.5–1.0 g IV, IM
- Pralidoxime methylsulphate   0.2–0.5 g IV, IM
- Obidoxime   0.25 g IV, IM
- Trimedoxime   0.2–0.25 g IV, IM
- Methoxime   1.0 g IV, IM
- HI-6   0.8–1.0 g IV

Figure 6.6 Recommended doses of reactivators for human use.

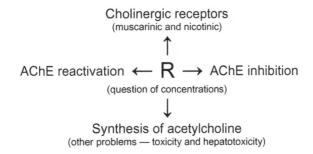

Cholinergic receptors
(muscarinic and nicotinic)

↑

AChE reactivation ← R → AChE inhibition

(question of concentrations)

↓

Synthesis of acetylcholine
(other problems — toxicity and hepatotoxicity)

Figure 6.7 Multiple effects of reactivators.

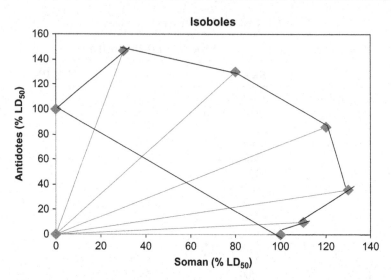

Figure 6.8 Method of isoboles. Combined lethal effect of soman in mice. Combination of soman (IM) and antidotes (atropin and obidoxime, IM, 2 min after the intoxication) in mice. 100% of LD_{50} = 148.8 mg/kg.

is expressing the affinity of the reactivator to the inhibited enzyme, and k_R is the velocity of its splitting. The second-order rate constant (k_r) represents the overall reactivation ability; it is calculated as the ratio (Equation 6.1):

$$k_r = k_R/K_R \tag{6.1}$$

The percentage of reactivation is calculated as the percentage of reactivation *in vitro* (Equation 6.2):

$$\%R = [1 - (a_0 - a_r)/(a_0 - a_i)] \times 100 \tag{6.2}$$

The reactivation (%) *in vivo* was determined by a similar approach using the AChE activity values (Equation 6.3):

$$\%R = [1 - (a_0 - a_r)/(a_0 - a_i)] \times 100 \tag{6.3}$$

where

a_o is activity in the control group (with administration of saline)
a_r is activity in the tabun-intoxicated group treated with atropine and reactivator
a_i is activity in the tabun-intoxicated group treated with atropine only.

The second-order rate constant of reactivation (k_r) is calculated using Equation 6.4:

$$k_r = k_R/K_R \tag{6.4}$$

Table 6.2 Reactivation Constants of Tabun-Inhibited AChE from Rat (R) and Human (H) Brain

Reactivator	Constant		
	K_R (μM)	k_R (min^{-1})	k_r (min^{-1}M^{-1})
K 203 (R)	6	0.096	16,000
K 203 (H)	56	0.120	2,142
Pralidoxime (R)	4,360	0.29	67
Pralidoxime (H)	2,810	0.19	68
Obidoxime (R)	2,450	0.12	49
Obidoxime (H)	144	0.03	208
HI-6 (R)	389	0.39	1,003
HI-6 (H)	181	0.08	441
K 027 (R)	54	0.0148	273
K 027 (H)	2,512	0.05	20
K 048 (R)	93	0.0324	348
K 048 (H)	251	0.06	239
Trimedoxime (H)	1,585	0.08	50
Methoxime (H)	2,512	0.05	20

Source: Different sources, mostly Kuca and Kassa (2003); Kuca et al. (2005, 2007a,b,c, 2011).

The dissociation constant (K_{diss}) can be obtained by nonlinear regression from the dependence of v on C_R using Equation 6.5:

$$v = v_{max} \times C_S/[C_S + K_M \times (1 + C_R/K_{diss})] \tag{6.5}$$

where v_{max} is the maximal (limiting) rate of the enzymatic reaction, C_S is the substrate concentration, and K_M is the Michaelis constant for the substrate used; e.g., for acetylcholine it is 1.9×10^{-4} M (Kassa and Cabal, 1999).

Reactivation constants for different reactivators and AChE inhibited by various nerve agents (OP) are in the literature. It is difficult to compare these constants; an illustration is given in Table 6.2. As the source of enzyme (AChE), human and rat brain homogenate was chosen. As inhibitor, tabun was chosen as a nerve agent. Tabun-inhibited AChE is reactivated by various reactivators differently and, for example, HI-6 is not an effective reactivator.

6.2 Development of New Reactivators

In the research of new cholinesterase reactivators, a complex approach was described by Kassa et al. (2007, 2012). The scheme in Figure 6.9 shows different steps of development and examination of new reactivators; it contains following steps: before synthesis, theoretical studies are performed: it is prediction of new structures using

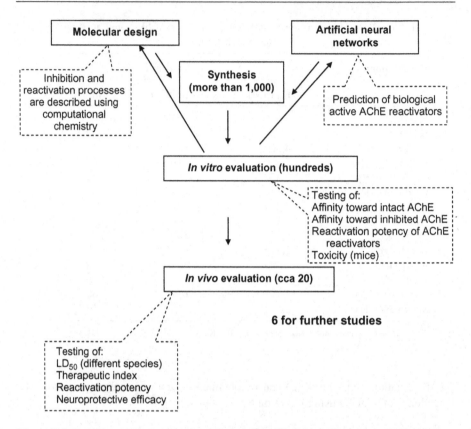

Figure 6.9 Developmental process of reactivators. Modified from Kassa et al. (2007, 2012).

artificial neuronal network (ANN), allowing to "learn" ANN without knowledge of exact interaction between a compound and an organism/biological system/enzyme. Thus, it is not necessary to synthesize the compound and it is possible to estimate biological activity. The part of these studies is also modeling of binding of oxime to AChE molecule. As an example, this binding of oximes on AChE is shown in Figure 6.10. Reactivators predicted by ANN and molecular design are synthesized; after synthesis, screening of AChE inhibition/reactivation (at two oxime concentrations: 10^{-5} and 10^{-3} M) are performed; sarin, tabun, soman, and cyclosarin are used for 95% AChE inhibition (up to now, more than 1,000 compounds have been tested). The next step is the study of inhibition/reactivation at the concentration ranging from 10^{-8} to 10^{-5} M (hundreds compounds). The kinetics (inhibition/reactivation) with four nerve agents and large scale of reactivator concentration is the next step; about 50 compounds are involved.

In vivo testing (toxicity in mice, rats, and guinea pigs; reactivation; therapeutic index and behavior) is followed (about 20 compounds). They are tested *in vitro* for reactivation efficacy with other nerve agents and OP insecticides (VX, dichlorvos, paraoxon).

At this step, antidotal efficacy on mice is determined; for antidotal treatment, the reactivator is combined with atropine (simultaneous administration 1 or 2 min

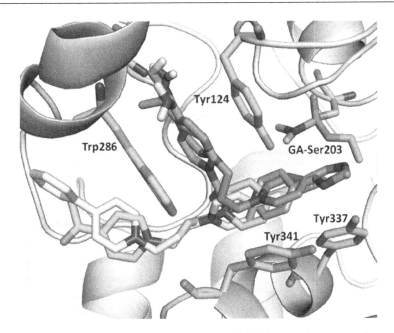

Figure 6.10 Top-scored docking poses of compounds K 027 (magenta), compound substituted with phenyl on pyridinium ring (yellow), compound substituted with COMet on pyridinium ring (blue) and compound substituted with $C(NH_2) = NOH$ on pyridinium ring (orange). (For interpretation of the references to color in this figure legend, the reader is referred to the web version of this book.)
Source: Reprinted with permission from Musilek et al. (2011).

after the intoxication, all IM administration). In the case of prophylaxis, antidotes are administered (IM) 10–20 min before the intoxication. The first nerve agent for prophylaxis is soman followed by VX, sarin, and others. The dose of reactivator is usually 10% of LD_{50} corresponding to the human dose and excluding possible inhibition effect of the reactivator at the higher doses (for both—either therapeutic or prophylactic effects). Inhibition or reactivation potency of the nerve agent or reactivator to AChE can be used to characterize the toxic effects (determination of cholinesterase activities in mice and rats). For the very promising oxime (approximately six compounds), further studies (plasma concentration, penetration of the blood–brain barrier, and others) are performed. The effect of various reactivators is different.

For example, from the historical point of view, pralidoxime is the first and most used AChE reactivator. However, the potency of pralidoxime to reactivate tabun-, cyclosarin-, soman-, or pesticide-inhibited AChE is not good enough. This is probably the reason for replacement of pralidoxime by methoxime in the US Army. In the literature, its use during pesticide poisoning was discussed many times. If pesticides are discussed, obidoxime and trimedoxime are the most promising reactivators. However, their potencies to reactivate cyclosarin- and soman-inhibited AChE are poor. If tabun-inhibited AChE reactivation is discussed, then these reactivators are promising compared with other commercially available ones. Another currently

Table 6.3 Comparison of Reactivation Effectiveness of Oximes HI-6 and HLö-7 (Two Concentrations) on AChE (Rat, Brain Homogenate) Inhibited by Different Nerve Agents *in vitro*

Nerve Agent (95% AChE inhibition)	HI-6/HLö-7 (10^{-5} M, % reactivation)	HI-6/HLö-7 (10^{-3} M, % reactivation)
Tabun	4/2	2/3
Sarin	49/7	47/25
Cyclosarin	28/24	52/31
Soman	16/24	23/86
VX	14/47	28/32
RVX	14/not tested	42/not tested

Source: According to Kuca et al. (2011).

available oxime on the market—methoxime—seems to be very promising in the case of cyclosarin, sarin, and VX poisoning. Its potency to reactivate tabun, soman, and pesticides poisoning is poor. The most promising oxime of commercially available ones is H-oxime HI-6. In view of military purposes (e.g., an antidote against nerve agents), it is able to reactivate almost all nerve agent-inhibited AChE with exception of tabun. On the contrary, if civilian importance is considered, HI-6 is unable to reactivate AChE in case of OP pesticide poisoning. From this very short summarization of antidotal effect of reactivators against nerve agent or OP poisoning, it is clear that there are relatively effective oximes (trimedoxime, obidoxime, methoxime), but the most effective seems to be the oxime HI-6. These observations are supported by extensive reviews dealing with the mentioned topics (Kassa, 2002; Kassa et al., 2012; Lundy et al., 2006).

There are other oximes slightly better than HI-6 (e.g., HLö-7), but preclinical and clinical research obligatory for their permission of clinical use and involvement into medical practice is expensive and final result (as therapeutic effectiveness) is not sufficient. The same can be applied for oximes K-048, K-027, K-203, and so on. The automatic administration of antidotes is solved by the use of autoinjector, but the question of content (effective antidotes) of autoinjector is more complicated.

As mentioned previously, HI-6 is very good reactivator; other oxime, HLö-7, is comparable with them but not significantly better. The differences in reactivation effectiveness of two prospective reactivators—HI-6 and HLö-7—are shown in Table 6.3.

6.3 Possibilities of AChE Reactivation

Comparison of AChE reactivatability of different oximes and various nerve agents *in vitro*—i.e., the dependence of the percentage of reactivation versus concentration of the oxime basically shows two different types of curves. Depending on the oxime concentration, the first demonstrates an increase with a maximum followed by a decrease. The second type is a sigmoid curve reaching to the maximum, but the decrease cannot

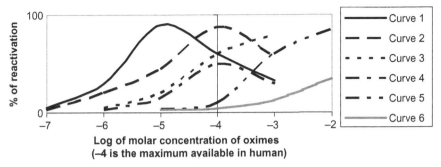

Figure 6.11 Hypothetic course of nerve agent–inhibited AChE reactivation by different oximes. Different curves represent the nerve agent–reactivator relationship. Curve 1—GF-methoxime, sarin-HI-6, HLö-7; curve 2—GF-HI-6; curve 3—soman-HI-6, HLö-7; curve 4—GF-HLö-7; curve 5—sarin-methoxime, pralidoxime, obidoxime; curve 6—soman-methoxime, pralidoxime, obidoxime, GF-pralidoxime, obidoxime.
Source: Reprinted from Bajgar (2004) with permission.

be demonstrated because the oxime concentration is too high (very probably it will be the same—i.e., containing a decreasing part). The first type can be represented by HI-6 and HLö-7 for sarin-inhibited AChE and methoxime and HI-6 for cyclosarin-inhibited AChE. HLö-7 has a similar profile in comparison with HI-6, but the AChE reactivation reaches to 50–60% only. For soman-inhibited AChE, HI-6 and HLö-7 show the second type of curve reaching the reactivation maximum at 10^{-4} to 10^{-5} M. Pralidoxime and methoxime show a similar profile; however, the lower reactivation (about 30–40%) was observed at the concentration 10^{-3} M. Obidoxime is ineffective in this case. Obidoxime and pralidoxime are effective against cyclosarin- and sarin-inhibited AChE at concentrations reaching to 10^{-3} to 10^{-2} M (Figure 6.11).

6.4   Available Concentrations of Oximes

The maximum concentration of oxime in the plasma after IM administration depends on its type and the dose administered. Relatively short half-lives were observed, depending on the type of organism. It reaches C_{max} in minutes (50–60min) lasting hours after the administration. For therapeutic action, it is essential to achieve the oxime concentration necessary for satisfactory reactivation in the target organs, especially in the brain. From different studies, it can be generally assessed that the oxime concentration in the plasma is approximately one-tenth of the administered dose. Its oral administration is not effective because of its quick degradation in the gastrointestinal tract.

The reactivator's effect on the CNS continues to be discussed. Because of their quaternary structure at intact blood–brain barrier, the penetration of reactivators is slow. The effectiveness of the oxime in humans can be influenced by the concentration in the target organs—i.e., when administered parenterally, in the dose range of 470–2,280 μmol/kg, the concentration in the brain can be about 10^{-4} to 10^{-5} M.

These concentrations are able to reactivate sufficiently inhibited AChE in the brain, especially in the pontomedullar area (a 10–20% increase): the minimal level of AChE activity in the pontomedullar area necessary for the survival of nerve agent–intoxicated animals was assessed to be about 5–20%. This concentration *in vitro* varies with the type of oxime used. In general, concentrations of 10^{-4} to 10^{-5} M can be considered as suitable for AChE reactivation *in vitro*, but at lower concentrations a small but significant reactivation also was observed.

Direct evidences for presence of oximes in the brain were demonstrated by Sakurada et al. (2003) using microdialysis detection of pralidoxime. A similar observation detecting AChE reactivation in the brain was described by others (Bajgar et al., 2010a; Kassa et al., 2012).

Concentrations of some oximes (e.g., HI-6, obidoxime, K-027, and K-048) in the rat plasma were determined, and it was assessed that concentration in the brain would be about 10^{-5} M (Kalasz et al., 2006; Karasova et al., 2011; Tekes et al., 2006). In this connection, special importance can be focused on the pontomedullar area where the respiration is regulated (Gupta, 2009) by cholinergic neurons (Kubin and Fenik, 2004; Sungur and Guven, 2001). Although homogenate reactivation in the whole brain was not observed (Kassa and Cabal, 1999), selective but not very high AChE reactivation was demonstrated in different brain parts, in particular the pontomedullar area (Bajgar et al., 2010a).

Thus, reactivators are able to penetrate the blood–brain barrier, and the published data demonstrate their reactivation effect in the brain. However, the reactivation effect is selective for different brain areas. This may be a reason for a false negative reactivation in the brain (the experiments were performed using the whole brain homogenate). When the sufficient AChE reactivation is present in physiologically important area, a good therapeutic effect was observed: survival of intoxicated animals correlated with the AChE activity in the pontomedullar area.

6.5   The Way to a Universal Oxime

There are two possibilities to obtain a universal reactivator:

1. Search for new oximes that are more effective with the aim of increasing their universality (current results did not show a universal oxime).
2. Use two (or more) oximes—their combinations—to cover all types of nerve agents and OPs.

Current studies did not show a universal oxime. There were some attempts to solve this problem using two oximes differently reactivating AChE inhibited by various nerve agents.

The effect of a combination of two reactivators was tested *in vitro* with obidoxime and HI-6 on AChE inhibited by tabun; it was demonstrated that the reactivating effect is the result of the effective oxime (i.e., obidoxime in case of tabun-inhibited AChE); the combination of obidoxime with HI-6 copied the effect of obidoxime alone (Worek et al., 2007). A similar combination (HI-6 and trimedoxime) was tested in rats *in vivo*; it was concluded that the AChE reactivation *in vivo* is not a summation (or simple copying) of the effect of a more effective oxime, but it is significantly higher (Bajgar et al., 2010c; Eyer, 2003; Kassa et al., 2007, 2012). The mechanism of this increase is necessary to elucidate in a more detailed way because other possibilities are not excluded: it is possible that the oximes blocked the AChE from phosphorylation by tabun or that its reactivation by trimedoxime is enhanced allosterically by HI-6. Perhaps interaction of AChE with tabun (slow) influences AChE activity so that it is a real chance to protect part of the enzyme. The affinity of HI-6 and trimedoxime to intact AChE supports this idea (see also Table 6.2). Moreover, AChE activity depends on the dose of oxime—its lower dose results in lower protection. Simultaneously, the toxicity of trimedoxime is higher than that of HI-6 (see also Table 6.1). Thus, it cannot be excluded that reactivation by trimedoxime and protection by HI-6 are combined. Different pharmacokinetics of oximes would not be a main reason for potentiation because the maximum concentration of oximes was achieved before the interval measured (Bajgar et al., 2010c).

However, a better therapeutic effect for two oximes was described independently, so one possible way to solve the problem of universal reactivator could be the use of two reactivators. When the combination of oximes is used for the treatment, the protective index is increased (Figure 6.12) and reactivation is also potentiated (Figure 6.13). For example, protective indexes in mice intoxicated with tabun and soman and treated with atropine and oxime alone or oxime combinations are higher than simple summation.

Reactivators alone are (in the absence of nerve agents) able to inhibit AChE of different sources; their affinity is different as documented in Table 6.4. However, there is no known detailed toxic mechanism of action of reactivators, although some biochemical parameters are clearly affected (Figure 6.14).

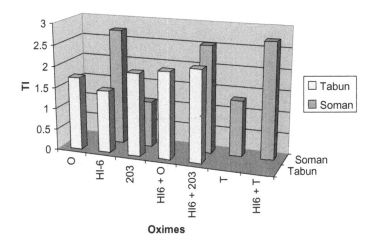

Figure 6.12 Protective indexes in mice intoxicated with tabun and soman and treated with atropine and oxime alone or oxime combinations.
Source: Modified from Kassa et al. (2012).

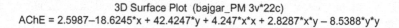

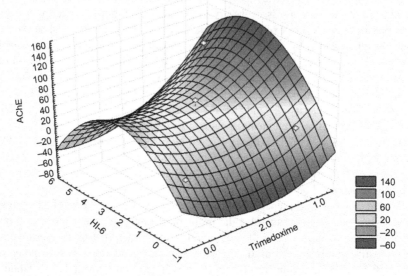

Figure 6.13 AChE reactivation in the pontomedullar area *in vivo* following tabun intoxication and its treatment.

Table 6.4 Affinities of Some Reactivators to the Recombinant Human AChE

Reactivator	IC_{50} (μM)
Pralidoxime	878
Obidoxime	577
Trimedoxime	167
Methoxime	2,010
HI-6	203
K-203	566
K-027	414

Source: Modified from Musilek et al. (2011).

6.6   Autoinjectors: Approach in Different Countries

It appears from the real threat of nerve agents that life-saving administration of antidotes is very topical. For the treatment, it was necessary to develop a drug-delivery device that allows minimally trained individuals to self-inject antidotes quickly before qualified medical treatment. The dose of administered antidote has to be precise to obtain maximum effectiveness. This military concept was applied for civilian use, too.

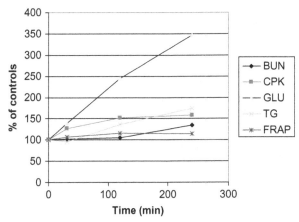

Figure 6.14 Changes in some biochemical parameters in dog following high dose of HI-6. *Source*: Modified from Pohanka et al. (2011).

Different approaches to the treatment of nerve agent poisoning were observed in different countries (the United States and Western and Eastern countries). Because of the very fast action of nerve agents, quick and easy injection of antidotes is necessary to increase the probability of survival. The devices that allow automatic administration of drugs by injection—autoinjectors—were developed (Atropen) in the United States in 1951. Other autoinjectors followed in many armies for first aid in the case of nerve agent exposure.

The father of the concept of the automatic syringe or autoinjector was Dr. S.J. Sarnoff (see Mesa, 2010). Technical possibilities changed over the years; the autoinjector has been in military use for more than 50 years. The first one was a laic injection syringe consisting of a tube filled with a drug and a needle. This syringe was kept in military stocks of many armies; Figure 6.15A demonstrates this device in the former Czechoslovakia. It was filled with atropine only. Then different concepts were developed—e.g., the autoinjector GAI (Figure 6.15B) was developed in the former East Germany and Czechoslovakia. Similar approaches were observed in Western countries. However, or equal or of even more importance is the content of an autoinjector containing atropine and a reactivator. For atropine, the dose is limited by its side effect; the dose of 2 mg seems to be as high as possible to begin therapeutic action and as low as possible to avoid side effects. The choice of reactivator is a more complicated question.

In the United States, where the autoinjector was first developed, pralidoxime was chosen as a reactivator. Its efficacy against nerve agents is not good enough, although it has remained in use by the US military up to now. Currently, it is considering replacement of pralidoxime for methoxime, but tests have not been finalized. The autoinjectors (a ComboPen with atropine and obidoxime) are now common in many armies (Figure 6.15C).

In Europe, probably in the light of the synthesis of H-oximes in Germany (and their significantly better reactivation effect), obidoxime was preferred. Autoinjectors containing atropine and obidoxime were in the equipment of European NATO

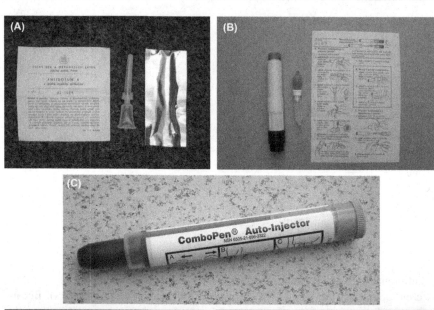

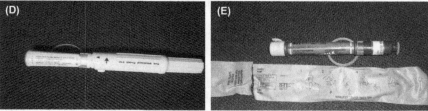

Figure 6.15 Different means for the first aid: (A) laic injection syringe, (B) autoinjector GAI, (C) an autoinjector ComboPen, (D) two-chambered autoinjector ASTRA, (E) two-chambered autoinjector STI.

countries as well as in former Warsaw Treaty countries. One small exception was the former USSR; antidotes were top secret. Moreover, the rules of permission in the former USSR were not comparable with the rest of the Eastern bloc (especially East Germany and Czechoslovakia): the tendency of these two countries was to have the autoinjector not only for military use but also available for civilian use. Therefore, it was necessary to perform all tests needed for permission in European Union countries. In the former USSR, many different antidotes were developed. However, in the absence of strict rules of their administration to healthy volunteers, it came up to side effects (perhaps a reason of secrecy). The detailed composition of Russian antidotes is unknown; generally, the antidotal mixture probably contains budoxime, two cholinolytics, atropine in lower dose, and an antioxidant.

Currently, generally two types of autoinjectors (with atropine and a reactivator) are mostly used. A ComboPen contains atropine and obidoxime in one solution; it is the first choice. However, the use of a more effective reactivator (HI-6) using this type of autoinjector is strictly limited because of the decomposition of HI-6 in solution. This situation can be solved using a wet and dry (two-chambered) autoinjector containing a solution of atropine in one chamber and the reactivator HI-6 in powdered (lyophilized) form (HI-6 chloride) in the second one. They are produced by ASTRA (Sweden) and STI (United States) (Figure 6.15D, E). The French bicompartment autoinjector was also demonstrated (Mendes-Oustric et al., 2006). When these autoinjectors are used, the content of the chambers is mixed and HI-6 is solubilized; the autoinjector needs to be shaken (5–10 s) before injection is needed.

There is only limited experience in human poisoning by highly toxic OP or nerve agents, but it is generally accepted that the persistence of clinically relevant amounts of nerve agent in blood is shorter than that of OPs. It is suggested that in the absence of clinical improvement, administration of oxime for periods in excess of 24–48 h is unlikely to achieve further reactivating of the enzyme (for review, see Kassa et al., 2011). Other studies of HI-6 in healthy volunteers (in combinations with atropine 2 mg) showed that changes observed following HI-6 treatment were not clinically important. HI-6 is involved in the equipment of the Czech, Slovak, Swedish, and Canadian armies as an antidote against nerve agent intoxication.

HI-6 in two-chambered autoinjectors is used as a chloride salt. Its physical and chemical properties are sufficient, but are other salts of HI-6 have these properties (especially solubility) more than chloride. The solubility of HI-6 dimethanesulfonate (HI-6 DMS) was much better in comparison with HI-6 chloride; this property is very useful for the use of HI-6 DMS in the autoinjector. Simultaneously, it was clearly demonstrated that the reactivation potency of HI-6 DMS in comparison with HI-6 chloride *in vitro* and *in vivo* was the same or better (Bajgar, 2009; Kuca et al., 2011). Thus, thanks to better solubility, it is clear that HI-6 DMS is more convenient for use as an antidote in the autoinjector against nerve agents.

6.7   Two- or Three-Chambered Autoinjector

Practical use of antidotes in the automatic devices is limited by the stability of the drug in solution contained in the autoinjector. Two autoinjectors for first aid against nerve agents are used in different armies: an autoinjector containing atropine and a reactivator (usually obidoxime) and an autoinjector with diazepam. It appears from previous analysis that the use of the better oxime—HI-6—is not applicable because of the low stability of HI-6 in solution. For the use of HI-6, a two-chambered autoinjector is necessary. The chambers contain atropine in solution and lyophylized HI-6 chloride. In all cases, it is one device for a soldier; the second one is another autoinjector for diazepam administration. Thus, two administrations (and two manipulations) are necessary for first aid. The idea of a three-chambered autoinjector is more interesting: the content of three-chambered autoinjector is atropine in solution, the best reactivator (HI-6) as a lyophilized powder, and diazepam in solution. For administration of all types of antidotes using three-chambered autoinjectors, one manipulation only is needed. Moreover, the content of the chambers can be changed according to proposed requirements—e.g., adding a new anticholinergic drug such as

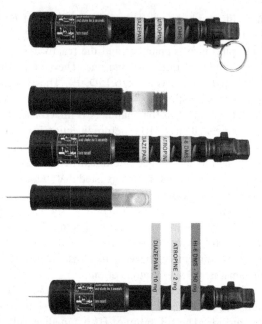

Figure 6.16 Three-chambered autoinjector. Produced by ChemProtect, Cukrovarnicka 62, 14200 Prague 6, www. chemprotect.eu

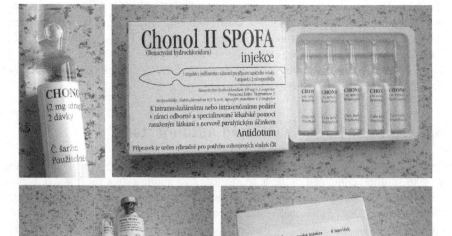

Figure 6.17 Multipacks of antidotes for medical treatment: anticholinergics—atropine (CHONOL I), benactyzine (CHONOL II); reactivators—methoxime (RENOL), HI-6 (ANTIVA).

Table 6.5 Possible Types of Antidotal Treatment of OP and Nerve Agent Intoxication, Including Problems and Their Solution

Type of Treatment	Main Problem	Solution	Practical Output
Atropine	Absence of central effects	For further treatment—central anticholinergics	CHONOL II (benactyzine, for medical treatment)
		Adding of reactivators	Autoinjector (atropine + obidoxime)
Reactivators	Isolated administration ineffective Methoxime DMS	Adding of anticholinergics Development (United States)	
Choice of reactivator	Absence of universal oxime	Use of present most effective oxime supplementary oxime	ANTIVA (HI-6, for medical treatment) RENOL (methoxime, for medical treatment)
Universal reactivator	Up to now unknown The choice of oximes	Further research Two reactivators	Three-chambered autoinjector
Reactivation of inhibited AChE	Route of administration	Transdermal	TRANSANT (HI-6 (also for prophylaxis)
Treatment convulsions (neuronal death)	Low efficacy	Further research	
Other compounds	Mechanism of action	Further research	

Source: Modified from Bajgar (2004, 2009), Gupta (2009), and Weissman and Raveh (2010).

benactyzine or akineton or centrally acting anticholinergic drugs with good antidotal effect against nerve agents such as soman. It does not exclude changing chamber contents by quite different drugs such as other benzodiazepines (e.g., midazolam) or other reactivators according to customer's request. In connection with nerve agent intoxication (especially tabun exposure), the autoinjector can be used also for prophylaxis, either with classic prophylactics as described or new ones (e.g., huperzine A); simultaneously, it could be of interest to replace diazepam with another reactivator. As previously mentioned, a universal reactivator has yet to be found. There were some attempts to solve this problem using two oximes that differentially reactivated AChE inhibited by various nerve agents.

Therefore, one possible way to obtain a universal reactivator would be to use two reactivators. A three-chambered autoinjector is the ideal device for this purpose (Figure 6.16). It is supposed that this autoinjector will be in the equipment of the Czech army. For medical treatment, there is a general precondition in many armies that repeated administration of the contents of an autoinjector (atropine and a reactivator) would be suitable, with other antidotes administered in hospital. However, in the Czech and Slovak armies, antidotes for medical treatment are involved as anticholinergics, a multipack of atropine for further atropinization (CHONOL I), and a multipack of benactyzine for treating central effects (CHONOL II) are available. Reactivators methoxime (RENOL) and HI-6 (ANTIVA) are contained in this equipment, too (Figure 6.17).

Some of the problems connected with the treatment of OP or nerve agent intoxication, including their solutions, are summarized in Table 6.5.

Conclusions

The treatment of nerve agent intoxication is based on good knowledge of pharmacodynamics; increased information of all these reactions in general will result in more effective therapy. Current antidotes comprise anticholinergics (preferably atropine), cholinesterase reactivators (different compounds), and anticonvulsants (diazepam). Currently, HI-6 can be considered as the optimal reactivator for the treatment of nerve agents' intoxication. Following administration of HI-6 to healthy volunteers, the changes observed are not of clinical importance. HI-6 DMS (lyophilized form) is more suitable for the use in the autoinjector than HI-6 dichloride. The three-chambered autoinjector can be considered the optimal device for administration of antidotes against nerve agent intoxication Development of other antidotes is in progress.

7 Prophylaxis

In general, the term prophylaxis can be characterized as a preventive measure against diseases or pathological change such as immunization or vaccination (against infectious diseases) or mechanical measures (e.g., the prevention of venereal diseases). It also comprises teeth cleaning (dental prophylaxis). From this point of view, decontamination of toxic chemicals is also prophylactic action, although it is not of a medical character and is an action taken before penetration of the toxic agent into the organism.

Prophylaxis against nerve agent intoxication means medical countermeasures applied relatively shortly before exposure or penetration of a toxic agent into the organism without further antidotal therapy. In the case of postexposure treatment, the administration of the drug before intoxication could be described as pretreatment. The term prophylaxis is limited to medical countermeasures applied relatively shortly before penetration of a toxic agent into the organism with the aim of protecting the organism against the toxic drug.

7.1 General Principles

Approaches to prophylaxis against nerve agents are based on different principles (Bajgar 2003, 2004; Bajgar et al., 2009; Gupta, 2009; Layish et al., 2005): keeping AChE intact (protection of AChE against inhibition) is a basic requirement for effective prophylaxis. This can be reached by using reversible inhibitors reversibly inhibiting AChE; it is resistant to OP or nerve agent inhibition. After spontaneous recovery of the activity (decarbamylation), normal AChE serves as a source of the active enzyme.

Detoxification can be used in two different ways: (1) administration of the enzymes splitting the OP and (2) evaluating specific enzymes bounded to the exogenously administered enzyme, thus decreasing the OP level in the organism (the so-called scavenger effect). The antidotes currently used for the treatment of OP poisoning can be tested as prophylactics. This principle can be considered as simulation of treatment or a treatment "in advance." Standard antidotes were studied in this respect—anticholinergics, reactivators, anticonvulsants, and others (Figure 7.1).

From the toxicodynamics of nerve agents, it appears that prophylactic countermeasures can bring two main actions: (1) protection of AChE against inhibition and (2) antagonization of the action of accumulated acetylcholine. In general, the protection of AChE against inhibition can be focused on the use of reversible cholinesterase inhibitors (preferably carbamates). Reversibly inhibited AChE by carbamates (carbamylated AChE) is resistant to OP or nerve agent inhibition effect. Carbamylated AChE is spontaneously decarbamylated and serves as a source of a native enzyme (Figure 7.2). Chemical structures of selected reversible inhibitors usable for prophylaxis are shown in Figure 7.3. Some of these compounds can be (or are) used for the treatment of Alzheimer's disease (e.g., Donepezil).

Nerve Agents Poisoning and its Treatment in Schematic Figures and Tables. DOI: 10.1016/B978-0-12-416047-7.00007-4

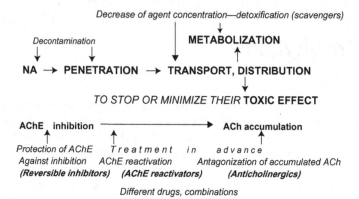

Figure 7.1 Schematic representation of basic toxicodynamic reactions during OP or nerve agent action and prophylactic countermeasures (in italics).
Source: Modified from Bajgar (2003), Bajgar et al. (2009), and Gupta (2009).

$$E + C \rightarrow EC \rightleftharpoons E + products$$
$$\uparrow \text{ not effective}$$
$$E + P \rightarrow EP1 \rightarrow EP2$$

Figure 7.2 Schematic representation of AChE protection using reversible inhibitors (carbamates). AChE (E) reacts with carbamate (C) to carbamylated enzyme (EC) and is spontaneously decarbamylated to normal AChE (E) and products. Carbamylated AChE is resistant to inhibition by OP or nerve agents (P). This reaction can be applied to other reversible inhibitors such as acridines.

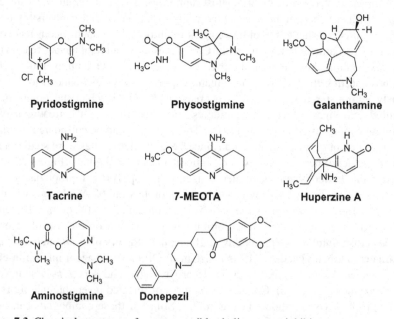

Pyridostigmine   Physostigmine   Galanthamine

Tacrine   7-MEOTA   Huperzine A

Aminostigmine   Donepezil

Figure 7.3 Chemical structures of some reversible cholinesterase inhibitors.

What happens during prophylaxis with reversible inhibitors? Briefly, following intoxication with nerve agent, a part of AChE is irreversibly inhibited in the central and peripheral nervous systems. Higher inhibition causes more pronounced symptoms that lead to death.

Following the administration of a reversible inhibitor, a part of AChE is reversibly inhibited (mostly carbamylated)—this part is resistant (protected) to the inhibition caused by the nerve agent or OP. It is spontaneously decarbamylated and forms normal AChE (serving as functional enzyme). A higher dose of reversible inhibitor leads to higher prophylactic efficacy (a higher amount of AChE is protected), but in the case of excessive inhibition, toxic signs (side effects) are manifested. Thus, the dosing of reversible inhibitor is a compromise between having the dose as high as possible for highest protection and as low as possible to minimize side effects. The most common inhibitor for prophylaxis is pyridostigmine. The administration of pyridostigmine as a prophylactic antidote is used in many armies. However, its inhibitory action is realized preferably in the peripheral nervous system. The dose of 30 mg PO 3 × daily is usual prophylactic intervention. An increased dose of reversible inhibitor without pronounced side effect can be solved by adding drugs that antagonize its toxic signs such as anticholinergics. Moreover, they are acting as therapeutic antidotes. This solution was used in the development of PANPAL (the original Czech prophylactic antidote). It is composed of pyridostigmine in higher dose (35 mg), and side effects are antagonized by administration of benactyzine (8 mg) and trihexyphenidyle (6 mg).

The presence of these two anticholinergics allowed us to increase the pyridostigmine dose and thus increase its prophylactic efficacy. This combination (including follow-up therapy) is not limited to soman, sarin, and VX poisoning, but its high efficacy against tabun and other nerve agents and some OPs was observed. The prophylactic combination PANPAL has no side effects as demonstrated on volunteers: no statistically different changes in the actual psychic state as well as the dysfunction time were observed. An improvement in the tapping test following PANPAL administration was demonstrated. A decrease in heart rate 60 min following PANPAL administration, lasting 480 min and returning to normal values within 24 h, also was demonstrated (Fusek et al., 2007). On the basis of the results with the prophylactic efficacy of other carbamates, aminostigmine also seems to be very effective.

Other carbamates also have a good prophylactic efficacy, especially physostigmine (because of its central effect contrary to pyridostigmine). A human study with transdermal physostigmine suggests a serious interest in the prophylactic use of this drug. Mobam, aminophenols, some OPs, and decarboxyfuran were also experimentally considered as potential candidates for prophylaxis, but their prophylactic effects were lower in comparison with pyridostigmine.

Structurally different inhibitors from the carbamate and OP groups were also studied. From these compounds (preferably binding to the AChE anionic site), tacrine, 7-methoxytacrine (7-MEOTA), and huperzine A were considered and experimentally studied with respect to prophylaxis *in vitro* and *in vivo*. The most interesting results were obtained with huperzine A. Huperzine A was tested as a potential candidate against OP for its long-lasting efficacy and relatively low toxicity and more pronounced central effect. However, the obtained results do not support replacement of pyridostigmine by these drugs.

The inhibitory effectiveness of some compounds to AChE and BuChE is given in Table 7.1. Similar to the case of nerve agents, the results are very dependent on methodical details (enzyme source, other conditions, etc.), and comparison is difficult. The role also plays the character of inhibition.

In case of prophylaxis by scavengers, the situation is quite different: following administration of scavenger, the part of the agent is bound to or hydrolyzed by exogenic administered compound and excluded from following toxic action—the level of nerve agent penetrating to the target sites is reduced. Thus, the principle is detoxification.

This principle can be used in two different ways: administration of the enzymes hydrolyzing OPs (catalytic scavengers) and evaluating specific enzymes binding nerve agent or OP to cholinesterase (stoichiometric scavengers).

In stoichiometric scavengers, the enzyme of cholinesterase type is administered (and its level in the organism is artificially increased—see also Figure 5.17D), and nerve agent is bound to the exogenously administered enzyme, thus decreasing the level of nerve agent in the organism (the scavenger effect). Enzymes hydrolyzing OPs or nerve agents—catalytic scavengers—are displaying a turnover with OPs or nerve agents as substrates, allowing rapid and efficient protection (Ditargiani et al., 2010; Masson et al., 1998). Paraoxonase seems to be very prospective (Aharoni et al., 2004; Rochu et al., 2008). On the other hand, many studies have been made with cholinesterases as scavengers. BuChE and AChE were observed to be very effective in protection against OP or nerve agent intoxication (Bajgar et al., 2009; Clark et al., 2002; Doctor et al., 1997; Gupta, 2009; Saxena et al., 2004). The administration of enzymes as scavengers seems to be very perspective: the enzyme is acting at very beginning of toxic action without interaction with target tissues and without side effects (Clark et al., 2002; Doctor et al., 1997). All of these features are of great interest and are leading to practical results (Huang et al., 2007; Saxena et al., 2004). There

Table 7.1 Constants IC_{50} (μM) for AChE (Enzyme Source—if Known in Parenthesis) and Other Organophosphorus Inhibitors

Compound	IC_{50} AChE (μM)	IC_{50} BuChE (μM)
Pyridostigmine	40 (human recombinant)	16,000 (human recombinant)
DMC	0.0016 (rat brain)	28 (horse plasma)
Tacrine	0.093 (rat cortex); 0.03; 2 4 (different); 4.0 (human)	0.074 (rat serum); 0.128; 1.0 (human)
7-MEOTA	3.63 (rat brain)	0.38 (rat plasma)
Physostigmine	0.15; 6.45; 0.012; 0.251 (rat cortex); 0.1819; 0.07; 0.6 (rat brain); 0.004 (human)	1.0; 0.035; 1.26 (rat serum); 0.07 (human)
Galantamine	1.995 (rat cortex)	12.59 (rat serum)
Donepezil	0.01 (rat cortex); 0.033; 0.014 (human)	5.01 (rat serum); 0.125; >100 (human)
Huperzine A	0.082 (rat cortex); 0.087 (rat erythrocytes); 0.3; 0.122	74.73 (rat serum); 117.3 (horse serum); 1259 (human serum)

Source: According to different references.

are problems with a lack of response and an autoimmune response and establishment of pharmacokinetic and pharmacodynamic properties. Recombinant human BuChE can be produced from the milk of transgenic goats (Cerasoli et al., 2005). Moreover, BuChE pretreatment also showed protective effects on AChE inhibition in the brain parts following low-level sarin inhalation exposure (Sevelova et al., 2004). There is a tendency to obtain a modified enzyme both splitting OP and simultaneously reacting with AChE as scavenger.

Simultaneous administration of BuChE and reactivators is also an interesting approach to prophylaxis: BuChE acts as a scavenger binding the nerve agent. A reactivator acting as a pseudocatalytic bioscavenger reactivates BuChE simultaneously, and the reactivated enzyme serves as a new scavenger (Jun et al., 2008).

Further studies show the best broad spectrum of AChE reactivators: trimedoxime and obidoxime in the case of paraoxon, leptophos-oxon, and methamidophos-inhibited AChE. In the case of BuChE, no reactivator exceeded 15% reactivation ability, and therefore none of the oximes can be recommended as a candidate for pseudocatalytic bioscavengers with BuChE (Jun et al., 2011).

Currently used antidotes also can be considered and tested as prophylactics. The problem of their use is timing, duration, and achievement of sufficient levels of these antidotes after the administration. The prolongation of the duration of an antidote's effect by achievement of sufficient levels in the blood by oral administration is not possible (especially reactivators) and therefore is excluded. Transdermal administration of one of the most effective reactivators (HI-6) was shown as the most realistic result in new prophylactic transdermal antidote TRANSANT (Bajgar, 2004, 2009, 2010c; Bajgar et al., 2004a, 2009; Fusek et al., 2007). It was clinically tested (including for dermal sensitivity) without any harmful effects. Field testing was also successful, and TRANSANT was introduced into the Czech army. Transdermal administration is very prospective. There are examples in clinical practice: transdermal scopolamine for the prevention of operative nausea and vomiting (not for prophylaxis); the study of hyoscine as a prophylactic drug; testing of transdermal physostigmine; and sustained release of physostigmine in combination with scopolamine (against side effects of physostigmine) (Meshulam et al., 2001). Prophylactic efficacy of other drugs also was studied. Anticonvulsants such as benzodiazepines (diazepam, midazolam, alprazolam, triazolam, clonazepam) were also studied but without good effects. For orientation, toxicities of different prophylactics or therapeutics are given in Table 7.2.

Summarizing the results dealing with prophylactic effect, the following drugs were tested as potential prophylactics: pyridostigmine, aminostigmine, physostigmine, huperzine A, acridines—7-MEOTA and tacrine from the group of reversible cholinesterase inhibitors; benactyzine, biperidene, scopolamine, atropine, and trihexyphenidyle from the group of anticholinergics; HI-6, 2-PAM, obidoxime, trimedoxime, and methoxime from the group of reactivators. Suramine, benzodiazepines, memantine, procyclidine, nimodipin, and clonidine are among other drugs tested. AChE, BuChE, mutants, triesterase, and paraoxonase are other prophylactics based on enzymatic nature. The search for catalytic bioscavenger continues (Ditargiani et al., 2010). Moreover, some prophylactic countermeasures can be applied for the

Table 7.2 Toxicities of Some Prophylactics or Therapeutics Against Nerve Agent Intoxication

Compound	Toxicity, IM (LD_{50}, mg/kg)		
	Mice	Rats	Other
Atropine	421	995–1264	Guinea pig, IV 163
	IV 74, PO 30–75	IV 117.4, PO 550	
Benactyzine	135–153	187.4	
		IV30.6	
Galantamine	6.8	24.3	
	IV 5.2, PO 18.7		
Pyridostigmine	3.08	2.79–8.22	
		SC11.0	
Physostigmine	0.86	2.2	Rabbit PO 11.2
	IP1.0		
Tacrine	28.9	33.8	
7-MEOTA	125	258	Dog IM 18.9
TrHPh	343.3	141.2	
	PO866.3		
Huperzine A	5.2	25.9	
	IV 0.63, IP 1.8	IV 2.55, IP 5.0	
Biperidene	545		
	IV 56		

treatment of nerve agent poisoning (Masson, 2011). Table 7.3 summarizes drugs used for prophylaxis.

Though the choice of prophylactics is relatively large, a small number of prophylactic drugs were chosen for medical military practice. The problems and their solutions in the research of prophylactics are shown in Table 7.4.

7.2 Prophylactics in Practice

Comparison of different prophylactic approaches to the rat model for pyridostigmine bromide, PANPAL, TRANSANT, and Protexia is given in Figure 7.4. Prophylactic antidotes PANPAL and TRANSANT are given in Figure 7.5.

Currently, PYRIDOSTIGMINE seems to be a common prophylactic antidote; PANPAL (tablets with pyridostigmine, trihexyphenidyle, and benactyzine) and TRANSANT (a transdermal patch containing HI-6) are other means introduced into different armies as prophylactics. Future development will be focused on scavengers (cholinesterases and other enzymes) acting before the binding of nerve agent to the target sites and to other drugs as either reversible cholinesterase inhibitors (e.g., huperzine A, physostigmine, and acridine derivatives) or other compounds.

These and many other studies were performed to improve prophylaxis of nerve agent or OP poisoning. This approach could lead to improvements in our knowledge

Table 7.3 Drugs Used in the Prophylaxis Against OP Poisoning

Principle	Drug Group	Drug	Duration	Equipment of the Army	Efficacy	Comment
Protection of cholinesterase inhibition	Carbamates	Pyridostigmine, aminostigmine, physostigmine Syntostigmine, eptastigmine, mobam Decarbofuran, heptylphosostigmine	8 h	Pyridostigmine bromide	+ + +	Dose limited, side effects Alone is not very effective, following antidotal treatment enhances its effect
	Others	**Huperzine A** Tacrine, methoxytacrine				
	OPs	TEPP, paraoxon Ethyl-4-nitrophenylphosphonate				
	Aminophenols	Eseroline				
Simulation of treatment	Anticholinergics	Biperidene, scopolamine, benactyzine Atropine, aprophen, hyoscine Adiphenine, caramiphen Pentamethonium, mecamylamine Trihexyphenidyle	8 h	TRANSANT (HI-6, transdermal administration)	+	Alone is not effective
	Reactivators	**HI-6** PAM, obidoxime, trimedoxime Methoxime				
	Others	**Suramine** Benzodiazepines, tubocurarine Memantine, procyclidine Nimodipin, clonidine				

(Continued)

Table 7.3 (Continued)

Principle	Drug Group	Drug	Duration	Equipment of the Army	Efficacy	Comment
Detoxification	**Cholinesterases** Enzymes hydrolyzing OP Monoclonal antibodies against OP	**Butyrylcholinesterase, mutants** AChE Triesterase Paraoxonase				Very perspective
Combinations			24 h? 8 h	Four combinations? PANPAL (pyridostigmine, trihexyphenidyle, benactyzine)	+ + + +? + + + +	No sufficient information Efficacy is increased with following antidotal treatment
				PANPAL + TRANSANT	+ + + + +	In combination, the best prophylactic efficacy

Source: Modified from Gupta (2009) with permission.
Relatively perspective drugs are in bold.

Table 7.4 Possible Types of Prophylaxis Against OP or Nerve Agent Intoxication Including Problems and Their Solving

Type of Prophylaxis	Main Problem	Solution	Practical Output
Reversible AChE inhibition	Side effects	Lower dose of pyridostigmine	PYRIDOSTIGMINE
		Adding of anticholinergics	PANPAL
Antagonisation of high acetylcholine level	Isolated administration limits prophylactic effect	Adding of reversible inhibitors	
Decrease of OP level stoichiometric scavengers	Immunologic reactions	PAGylation, purity, production, further research, suitable enzyme	Protexia®
Catalytic scavengers	Increase of catalytic activity		
Reactivation of inhibited AChE	Route of administration	Transdermal	TRANSANT
Antagonisation of convulsions	Low prophylactic efficacy	Further research	
Other compounds	Mechanism of action	Further research	

Source: Modified from Bajgar (2003, 2004), Bajgar et al. (2004a, 2009), and Gupta (2009).

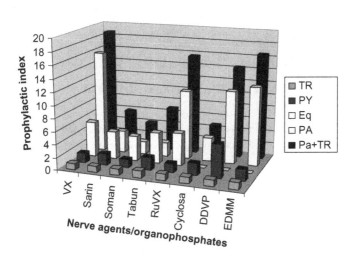

Figure 7.4 Prophylactic efficacy of different prophylactics against nerve agents or OPs in rats. The results are means only. TR = TRANSANT, PY = pyridostigmine, Eq = equine butyrylcholinesterase, PA = PANPAL, Pa + TR = combination of PANPAL and TRANSANT.
Source: According to Bajgar et al. (2010b).

(A)

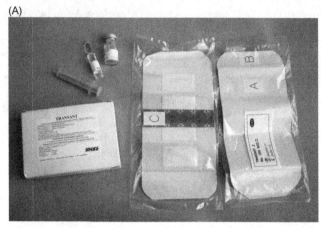

(B)

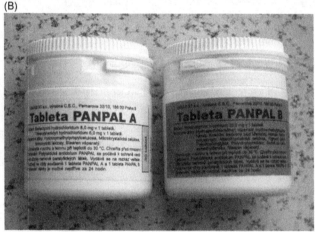

Figure 7.5 Prophylactic means (A) TRANSANT and (B) PANPAL.

of mechanisms of action of nerve agents and other inhibitors and to better therapeutic or prophylactic efficacy of the poisoning caused by these chemicals. Simultaneously, it could contribute to better understanding of cholinergic nerve transmission and thus to biochemistry, pharmacology, and neuropharmacology in general.

Conclusions

Prophylaxis is an important part of preventive measures against nerve agent poisoning. There are different approaches, but practical output is not currently good enough. For further development, it is necessary to search for new prophylactic drugs and new routes of administration. In this connection, preparations of cholinesterases are of special importance for the development of more effective prophylactics.

8 Conclusions

The mechanism of action of OPs or nerve agents needs to be studied in more detail, including not only cholinergic but also other neurotransmitter system changes, with the aim of preventing neuronal death from intensive seizures.

It is important to continue studying the binding of different ligands to the molecules of AChE and BuChE, including their molecular forms and receptors, with the aim of elucidating cholinergic nerve transmission, and on that basis improve prophylaxis and treatment of nerve agent poisoning. In connection with nonspecific effects, prospective drugs need to be experimentally tested.

Elucidating long-term effects is important for obtaining more information dealing with the effect of low doses (concentrations) of OPs or nerve agents and prophylactic or therapeutic countermeasures.

The gene expression profile after OP or nerve agent intoxication is important for the development of mechanism-based therapies and should be considered.

It is necessary to study the relationship between cholinesterases and their functions, including their changes in pathological states.

For actual treatment of acute intoxication, the choice of optimal reactivators and parasympatholytics as well as their timing is very important. Studying all countermeasures for the improvement of the state of organism intoxicated (e.g., pH changes, O_2, and CO_2 saturation) should be continued.

The synthesis of new reactivators using molecular modeling with the aim of obtaining universal reactivator also needs to be continued. However, universal reactivators (reactivating cholinesterases inhibited by all OPs or nerve agents) currently is probably a dream.

The use of more reactivators to improve treatment of OP or nerve agent poisoning needs further study.

To elucidate another than reactivation effect of oximes, including acute mechanism of toxic action needs more complex studies.

Improvement of prophylaxis using bioscavengers (both catalytic and stoichiometric) also needs further study. In this connection, the use of BuChE and its reactivation for prophylactic purposes should be examined.

New drugs for prophylaxis should be synthesized and tested, and combinations of scavengers and classic prophylactics should be developed.

Nerve Agents Poisoning and its Treatment in Schematic Figures and Tables. DOI: 10.1016/B978-0-12-416047-7.00008-6

References

Aharoni, A., Gaidukov, L., Yagur, S., Toker, L., Silman, I., Tawfik, D.S., 2004. Directed evolution of mammalian paraoxonases PON1 and PON3 for bacterial expression and catalytic specialization. Proc. Natl. Acad. Sci. U.S.A. 101, 482–487.

Allon, N., Rabinovitz, I., Manistersky, E., Weissman, B.A., Grauer, E., 2007. Acute and long-lasting cardiac changes following a single whole-body exposure to sarin vapor in rats. Toxicol. Sci. 87, 385–390.

Bajgar, J., 1991. The influence of inhibitors and other factors on cholinesterases. Sbor. Ved. Praci LF UK (Hradec Kralove) 34, 3–75.

Bajgar, J., 2003. Prophylaxis against organophosphorus poisoning. J. Med. Chem. Def. 1, 1–15.

Bajgar, J., 2005. Laboratory diagnosis of organophosphates/nerve agent poisoning. Klin. Biochem. Metab. 13, 40–47.

Bajgar, J., Voicu, V., 2009. Assessment of effective dose of nerve agents following different routes of administration. Therap. Pharmacol. Clin. Toxicol. 13, 131–138.

Bajgar, J., Fusek, J., Sevelova, L., Kassa, J., 2004a. Original transdermal prophylactic antidote against nerve agents—TRANSANT. CB Medical Treatment Symposium, 25–30 April 2004, Spiez, Switzerland, Technical Program, p. 14.

Bajgar, J., Sevelova, L., Krejcova, G., Fusek, J., Vachek, J., Kassa, J., et al. 2004b. Biochemical and behavioral effects of soman vapors in low concentrations. Inh. Toxicol. 16, 497–507.

Bajgar, J., Hajek, P., Slizova, D., Krs, O., Fusek, J., Kuca, K., et al. 2007. Changes of acetylcholinesterase activity in different brain areas following intoxication with nerve agents: biochemical and histochemical study. Chem. Biol. Interact. 165, 14–21.

Bajgar, J., Fusek, J., Kassa, J., Kuca, K., Jun, D., 2009. Chemical aspects of pharmacological prophylaxis against nerve agent poisoning. Curr. Med. Chem. 16, 2977–2986.

Bajgar, J., Hajek, P., Zdarova Karasova, J., Kassa, J., Paseka, A., Slizova, D., et al. 2010a. A comparison of tabun-inhibited rat brain acetylcholinesterase reactivation by three oximes (HI-6, obidoxime, and K048) in vivo detected by biochemical and histochemical techniques. J. Enz. Inh. Med. Chem. 25, 790–797.

Bajgar, J., Kassa, J., Fusek, J., Bartosova, L., 2010b. Comparison of different approaches to prophylaxis against nerve agents and organophosphates incidents. The Eighth International Chemical and Biological Medical Treatment Symposium, 2–7 May 2010, Spiez, Switzerland, Technical Program, Abstract No. 4, p. 20.

Bajgar, J., Zdarova Karasova, J., Kassa, J., Cabal, J., Fusek, J., Blaha, V., et al. 2010c. Tabun-inhibited rat tissue and blood cholinesterases and their reactivation with the combination of trimedoxime and HI-6. Chem.-Biol. Interact. 187, 287–290.

Bartosova, L., Kuca, K., Kunesova, G., Jun, D., 2006. The acute toxicity of acetylcholinesterase reactivators in mice in relation to their structure. Neurotoxicity Res. 9, 291–296.

Benschop, H.P., de Jong, L.P.A., 2001. Toxicokinetics of nerve agents. In: Somani, S.M., Romano, J.A. (Eds.), Chemical Warfare Agents: Toxicity at Low Levels. CRC Press, Boca Raton, FL, pp. 25–81.

Bloch-Shilderman, E., Levy, A., 2007. Transient and reversible nephrotoxicity of sarin in rats. J. Appl. Toxicol. 27, 189–194.

Bosak, A., Katalinic, M., Kovarik, Z., 2011. Cholinesterases: structure, role, and inhibition [in Croatian]. Arch. Indust. Hyg. Toxicol. 62, 175–190.

Cabal, J., Bajgar, J., Kassa, J., 2010. Evaluation of flow injection analysis for determination of cholinesterase activities in biological material. Chem. Biol. Interact. 187, 225–228.

Cerasoli, D.M., Griffiths, E.M., Doctor, B.P., Saxena, A., Fedorko, J.M., Greig, N.H., et al. 2005. In vitro and in vivo characterization of recombinant human butyrylcholinesterase (Protexia) as a potential nerve agent bioscavenger. Chem. Biol. Interact. 157, 363–365.

Clark, M.G., Saxena, A., Anderson, S.M., Sun, W., Bansal, R., et al., 2002. Behavioral toxicity of purified human serum butyrylcholinesterase in mice. Fourth International CBMTS, 28 April to 3 May 2002, Spiez, Switzerland, Abstract No. 19.

Collombet, J.M., 2011. Nerve agent intoxication: recent neuropathophysiological findings and subsequent impact on medical management prospects. Toxicol. Appl. Pharmacol. 255, 229–241.

Ditargiani, R.C., Chandrasekaran, L., Belinskaya, T., Saxena, A., 2010. In search of a catalytic bioscavenger for the prophylaxis of nerve agent toxicity. Chem. Biol. Interact. 187, 349–354.

Doctor, B.P., Maxwell, D.M., Saxena, A., 1997. Preparation and characterization of bioscavengers for possible use against organophosphate toxicity. M-CB Medical Treatment Symposium, 26–30 May 1997, Hradec Kralove, Czech Republic, Abstracts, pp. 17–18.

Du, D., Wang, J., Smith, J.N., Timchalk, C., Lin, Y., 2009. Biomonitoring of organophosphorus agent exposure by reactivation of cholinesterase enzyme based on carbon nanotube-enhanced flow-injection amperometric detection. Analyt. Chem. 81, 9314–9320.

Ellman, G.L., Courtney, D.K., Andres, V., Featherstone, R.M., 1961. A new and rapid colorimetric determination of acetylcholinesterase activity. Biochem. Pharmacol. 7, 88–95.

Eyer, P., 2003. The role of oximes in the management of organophosphorus pesticides poisoning. Toxicol. Rev. 22, 165–190.

Fidder, A., Hulst, A.G., Noort, D., de Ruiter, R., van der Schans, M.J., Benschop, H.P., et al. 2002. Retrospective detection of exposure to organophosphorus anti-cholinesterases: mass spectrometric analysis of phosphylated human butyrylcholinesterase. Chem. Res. Toxicol. 15, 582–590.

Fusek, J., Bajgar, J., Merka, V., 2007. Medikamentose prophylaxe bei vergiftungen mit nervenkampfstoffen. Koord. Sanitatsdienst 25, 41–47.

Gopalakrishnakone, P., 2003. Microarray analysis of the human brain cell lines following exposure to a chemical agent, soman. In: K. Laihia (Ed.), Symposium Proceedings NBC 2003, Javaskyla, pp. 146–147.

Gupta, R.C., 2004. Brain regional heterogenity and toxicological mechanisms of organophosphates and carbamates. Toxicol. Mech. Meth. 14, 103–143.

Huang, Y.-J., Huang, Y., Baldassarre, H., Wang, B., Lazaris, A., Leduc, M., et al. 2007. Recombinant human butyrylcholinesterase from milk of transgenic animals to protect against organophosphate poisoning. Proc. Natl. Acad. Sci. U.S.A. 104, 13603–13608.

Jokanovic, M., 2009. Current understanding of the mechanisms involved in metabolic detoxification of warfare nerve agents. Toxicol. Lett. 188, 1–10.

Jun, D., Musilova, L., Kuca, K., Kassa, J., Bajgar, J., 2008. Potency of several oximes to reactivate human acetylcholinesterase and butyrylcholinesterase inhibited by paraoxon in vitro. Chem. Biol. Interact. 175, 421–424.

Jun, D., Musilova, L., Musilek, K., Kuca, K., 2011. In vitro ability of currently available oximes to reactivate organophosphate pesticide-inhibited human acetylcholinesterase and butyrylcholinesterase. Internat. J. Mol. Sci. 12, 2077–2087.

Kalasz, H., Hasan, M.Y., Sheen, R., Kuca, K., Petroianu, G., Ludanyi, K., et al. 2006. HPLC analysis of K-48 concentration in plasma. Analyt. Bioanalyt. Chem. 385, 1062–1067.

Karasova Zdarova, J., Novotny, L., Antos, K., Zivna, H., Kuca, K., 2010. Time-dependent changes in concentration of two clinically used acetylcholinesterase reactivators (HI-6 and obidoxime) in rat plasma determined by HPLC techniques after *in vivo* administration. Analyt. Sci. 26, 63–67.

Karasova, J.Z., Zemek, F., Bajgar, J., Vasatova, M., Prochazka, P., Novotny, L., et al. 2011. Partition of bispyridinium oximes (trimedoxime and K074) administered in therapeutic doses into different parts of the rat brain. J. Pharm. Biomed. Anal. 54, 1082–1087.

Kassa, J., 2002. Review of oximes in the antidotal treatment of poisoning by organophosphorus nerve agents. J. Toxicol. Clin. Toxicol. 6, 803–816.

Kassa, J., Cabal, J., 1999. A comparison of the efficacy of a new asymmetric bispyridinium oxime BI-6 with currently available oximes and H oximes against soman by *in vitro* and *in vivo* methods. Toxicology 32, 11–118.

Kassa, J., Kuca, K., Karasova, J., Musilek, K., Jun, D., Bajgar, J., et al., 2007. Development of new reactivators of tabun-inhibited acetylcholinesterase and the evaluation of their efficacy by *in vitro* and *in vivo* methods. HFM-149 Symposium "Defense against the effects of chemical toxic hazards: Toxicology, diagnosis, and medical countermeasures." Edinburgh, Scotland (GBR), 8–10 October 2007, Session 4, OP Medical Countermeasures, No. 17.

Kassa, J., Musilek, K., Karasova, J.K., Kuca, K., Bajgar, J., 2012. Two possibilities how to increase the efficacy of antidotal treatment of nerve agent poisoning. Mini Rev. Med. Chem., 12, 24–34.

Kubin, L., Fenik, V., 2004. Pontine cholinergic mechanisms and their impact to respiratory regulation. Resp. Physiol. Neurobiol. 143, 235–249.

Kuca, K., Kassa, J., 2003. A comparison of the ability of a new bispyridinium oxime 1-(4-hydroxyiminomethylpyridinium)-4-(4-carbamoylpyridinium)butane dibromide and currently used oximes to reactivate nerve agent-inhibited rat brain acetylcholinesterase by *in vitro* methods. J. Enz. Inhib. Med. Chem. 18, 529–535.

Kuca, K., Bartosova, L., Jun, D., Patocka, J., Cabal, J., 2005. New quaternary pyridine aldoximes as causal antidotes against nerve agents intoxications. Biomed. Papers 149, 75–82.

Kuca, K., Cabal, J., Jun, D., Musilek, K., 2007a. *In vitro* reactivation potency of acetylcholinesterase reactivators—K074 and K075—to reactivate tabun inhibited human brain acetylcholinesterase. Neurotox. Res. 11, 101–106.

Kuca, K., Jun, D., Cabal, J., Musilova, L., 2007b. Bisquaternary oximes as reactivators of tabun-inhibited human brain cholinesterases: an *in vitro* study. Basic Clin. Pharmacol. Toxicol. 101, 25–28.

Kuca, K., Jun, D., Musilek, K., Bajgar, J., 2007c. Reactivators of tabun-inhibited acetylcholinesterase: structure–biological activity relationship. Fron. Drug Design Discov. 3, 381–394.

Kuca, K., Musilek, K., Karasova, J., Jun, D., Soukup, O., Pohanka, M., et al. 2011. On the universality of oxime HLo-7—antidote for case of the nerve agents poisoning. Mil. Med. Sci. Lett. (formerly Voj. Zdrav. Listy) 80, 80–84.

Layish, I., Krivoy, A., Rotman, E., Finkelstein, A., Tashma, Z., Yehezkelli, Y., 2005. Pharmacologic prophylaxis against nerve agent poisoning. Israel Med. Assoc. J. 7, 182–187.

Lundy, P.M., Raveh, L., Amitai, G., 2006. Development of the bisquaternary oxime HI-6 toward clinical use in the treatment of organophosphate nerve agent poisoning. Toxicol. Rev. 26, 231–243.

Masson, P., 2011. Evolution of and perspectives on therapeutic approaches to nerve agent poisoning. Toxicol. Lett. 206, 5–13.

Masson, P., Josse, D., Lockridge, O., Viguie, N., Taupin, C., Buhler, C., 1998. Enzymes hydrolyzing organophosphates as potential catalytic scavengers against organophosphate poisoning. J. Physiol. 92, 357–362.

Massoulié, J., Pezzementi, L., Bon, S., Krejci, E., Vallette, F.M., 1993. Molecular and cellular
biology of cholinesterases. Progr. Neurobiol. 41, 31–91.

Mendes-Oustric, C., Bardot, S., Clair, P., Lallement, G., Zabé, D., Renaudeau, C., 2006. The
bi-compartment auto-injector of the French military health service for emergency treatment of organophosphate poisoning. Sixty-Sixth International Congress of FIP Salvador
Bahia, 25–31 August 2006, Brazil.

Mesa, M., 2010. From battlefield to backpack: evolution of the autoinjector. ASA Newslett.
10-1 (136), 1, 15–18.

Meshulam, Y., Cohen, G., Chapman, S., Alkalai, D., Levy, A., 2001. Prophylaxis against organophosphate poisoning by sustained release of scopolamine and physostigmine. J. Appl.
Toxicol. 21 (Suppl. 1), S75–S78.

Musilek, K., Komloova, M., Holas, O., Horova, A., Pohanka, M., Gunn-Moore, F., et al. 2011.
Mono-oxime bisquaternary acetylcholinesterase reactivators with prop-1,3-diyl linkage –
preparation, in vitro screening and molecular docking. Bioorg. Med. Chem. 19, 754–762.

Noort, D., van der Schans, M.J., Bikker, F.J., Benschop, H.P., 2009. Diagnosis of exposure to chemical warfare agents: an essential tool to counteract chemical terrorism. In:
Dishovsky, C., Pivovarov, A. (Eds.), Counteraction to Chemical and Biological Terrorism
in East European Countries. Book Series: NATO Science for Peace and Security Series
A–Chemistry and Biology. Springer, Dordrecht, pp. 195–201.

Patocka, J. (Ed.), 2004. Military Toxicology [Vojenska toxikologie (in Czech)]. Grada-
Avicenum, Prague, 178 pp.

Pohanka, M., 2011. Cholinesterases: a target of pharmacology and toxicology. Biomed. Papers
155, 219–230.

Pohanka, M., Novotny, L., Zdarova-Karasova, J., Bandouchova, H., Zemek, F., Hrabinova,
M., et al. 2011. Asoxime (HI-6) impact on dogs after one and tenfold therapeutic doses:
assessment of adverse effects, distribution, and oxidative stress. Environ. Toxicol.
Pharmacol. 32, 75–81.

Rochu, D., Chabriere, E., Masson, P., 2008. Human paraoxonase: a promising approach
for pre-treatment and therapy of organophosphorus poisoning. Neurochem. Res. 33,
348–354.

Sakurada, K., Matsubara, K., Shimizu, K., Shiono, H., Seto, Y., Tsuge, K., et al. 2003.
Pralidoxime iodide (2-PAM) penetrates across the blood–brain barrier. Neurochem. Res.
28, 1401–1407.

Saxena, A., Doctor, B.P., Sun, W., Luo, C., Bansal, R., Naik, R.S., et al. 2004. HuBChE: a
bioscavenger for protection against organophosphate chemical warfare agents. U.S. Army
Medical Department J. 7, 22–29.

Sevelova, L., Bajgar, J., Saxena, A., Doctor, B.P., 2004. Protective effect of equine butyrylcholinesterase in inhalation intoxication of rats with sarin: determination of blood and brain
cholinesterase activities. Inhal. Toxicol. 16, 531–536.

Soukup, O., Tobin, G., Kumar, U.K., Binder, J., Proska, J., Jun, D., et al. 2010. Interaction of
nerve agent antidotes with cholinergic systems. Curr. Med. Chem. 17, 1708–1718.

Sprading, K.D., Lumley, L.A., Robison, C.L., Meyerhoff, J.L., Dillman, J.F., 2011.
Transcriptional responses to the nerve agent-sensitive brain regions amygdala, hippocam-
pus, pyriform cortex, septum, and thalamus following exposure to the organophosphonate
anticholinesterase sarin. J. Neuroinflam., 8.10.1186/1742-2094-8-84

Sungur, M., Guven, M., 2001. Intensive care management of organophosphate insecticide poisoning. Crit. Care 5, 211–215.

Tekes, K., Hasan, M.Y., Sheen, R., Kuca, K., Petroianu, G., Ludanyi, K., et al. 2006. High-performance liquid chromatographic determination of the plasma concentration of K-27, a novel oxime-type cholinesterase reactivator. J. Chromat. A 1122, 84–87.

Voicu, V., Bajgar, J., Medvedovici, A., Radulescu, F.S., Miron, D.S., 2010. Pharmacokinetics and pharmacodynamics of some oximes and associated therapeutic consequences: a critical review. J. Appl. Toxicol. 30, 719–729.

Wiesner, J., Kriz, Z., Kuca, K., Jun, D., Koca, J., 2007. Acetylcholinesterase: the structural similarities and differences. J. Enz. Inhib. Med. Chem. 22, 417–424.

Worek, F., Aurbek, N., Thiermann, H., 2007. Reactivation of organophosphate-inhibited human AChE by combinations of obidoxime and HI-6 *in vitro*. J. Appl. Toxicol. 27, 582–588.

Further reading

Aldridge, W.N., Reiner, E., 1973. Enzyme Inhibitors as Substrates. North Holland Publishing, Amsterdam, London.

Bajgar, J., 2004. Organophosphates/nerve agent poisoning: mechanism of action, diagnosis, prophylaxis, and treatmentMakowsky, G.M. Advances in Clinical Chemistry, vol. 38. Elsevier Academic Press, San Diego, CA, pp. 151–216.

Bajgar, J. (Ed.), 2009. Central and Peripheral Nervous System: Effects of Highly Toxic Organophosphates and Their Antidotes. Research Signpost, Kerala, India.

Fest, C., Schmidt, K.-J., 1982. The Chemistry of Organophosphorus Pesticides, 2nd rev. ed. Springer-Verlag, Berlin.

Gupta, R.C. (Ed.), 2006. Toxicology of Organophosphate and Carbamate Compounds. Elsevier/AP, Amsterdam.

Gupta, R.C. (Ed.), 2009. Handbook of Toxicology of Chemical Warfare Agents. Elsevier/AP, Amsterdam.

Koelle, G.B. (Ed.), 1963. Handbuch der experimentellen Pharmakologie. Cholinesterases and anticholinesterase agents. 15. Band. Springer-Verlag, Berlin.

Lenhart, M.K., Tuorinski, S.D. (Eds.), 2008. Textbooks in Military Medicine. Office of the Surgeon General, Department of the Army, United States of America and US Army Medical Department Center and School, Fort Sam Houston, San Antonia, TX.

Marrs, T.C., Maynard, R.L., Sidell, F.R., 1996. Chemical Warfare Agents Toxicology and Treatment. John Wiley & Sons, New York.

Romano Jr., J.A., Lukey, B.J., Salem, H. (Eds.), 2007. Chemical Warfare Agents: Chemistry, Pharmacology, Toxicology, and Therapeutics. CRC Press, Boca Raton, FL.

US Army Medical Research Institute of Chemical Defense, 2010. Medical Management of Chemical Casualties Handbook, third ed. US Army Medical Research Institute of Chemical Defense, Aberdeen, MD.

Weissman, B.A., Raveh, L. (Eds.), 2010. The Neurochemical Consequences of Organophosphate Poisoning in the CNS. Transworld Research Network, Kerala, India.

Printed in the United States
By Bookmasters